Grief Responses to Long-Term Illness and Disability

Grief Responses to Long-Term Illness and Disability

Manifestations and Nursing Interventions

EDITED BY

Jean A. Werner-Beland
Wayne State University

CONTRIBUTORS

Judith M. Agee
Wayne State University

Irene L. Beland
Wayne State University

Mary Delaney-Naumoff

E. Ingvarda Hanson
Wayne State University

Ann M. Zuzich
Wayne State University

RESTON PUBLISHING COMPANY, INC., Reston Virginia
A Prentice-Hall Company

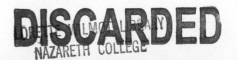

Library of Congress Cataloging in Publication Data

Main entry under title:

Grief responses to long-term illness and disability.

Includes bibliographies and index.
1. Nursing—Psychological aspects. 2. Grief.
3. Chronic diseases—Psychological aspects.
4. Physically handicapped—Psychology.
I. Werner-Beland, Jean A.
RT86.G74   155.9'16'024613   79-21452
ISBN 0-8359-2591-9 (C)
        0-8359- 2590- 0 (P)

© 1980 by Reston Publishing Company, Inc.
A Prentice-Hall Company
Reston, Virginia   22090

,7441°

10 9 8 7 6 5 4 3 2 1

Printed in the United States of America

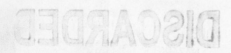

To all who help in so many ways,
in good times and in bad.

Contents

Preface, xi

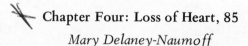

PART THREE

Chapter Seven: Nursing and the Concept of Hope, 169

Jean A. Werner-Beland

Chapter Eight: The Burnout Syndrome in Nurses, 189

Irene L. Beland

Preface

Multiple problems are faced by individuals, families, and caregivers who have contact with persons who have long-term illnesses or disabilities. One of these problems centers around the grief that is experienced, not only by the person who is ill or disabled, but also by others who are closely involved with this person. Grief responses are assumed to occur in all people who have severely altered body states as the result of illness or injury, but these responses are often ignored by nurses and other health professionals. Perhaps this is so because we are made anxious by anyone who poses a real or imagined threat to our own existence. Because dealing with the grieving patient poses so many problems, the aim here is to increase the nurse's understanding and ability to deal with grief responses in those who continue to live in spite of having suffered a severe assault to their physical well-being.

It is our contention that grief is a significant pivotal factor whose degree of resolution greatly influences the success or failure of many nursing efforts. This grief, and its manifest behaviors, frequently goes unrecognized or is little understood by those who are in a position to observe and help bring it to some degree of resolution. People in positions to observe the ill or disabled person need to be cognizant of the fact that grieving is a necessary concommitant of illness. However, grief also occurs in nonillness states, for example, as one ages or when one becomes the parent of a child with a birth defect. Specific chapters are devoted to these latter issues because it is our belief that it is not just the hospitalized patient who makes up the practice domain of nursing. Nursing, as we view it, has a responsibility to prevent illness or human suffering wherever possible; whether that be with the individual, the family, or the community.

Nurses who care for persons with long-term illnesses or disabilities may recognize what is happening with these persons and their significant others. As health professionals and concerned human beings, nurses themselves often have a high degree of emotional investment in their patients or clients. However, nurses also lack the support systems that would enable them to deal effectively with patients and families who are experiencing grief in response to physical illness. Nurses, in order to use their full human potential in helping others to deal with difficult emotional states, must realize that they are professionally ineluctably interdependent. Nurses must also realize that patients share this same interdependence in life, and this is no less true during the process of grief resolution and redefinition of self than at other times.

In addition to looking at the grief response in patients and their significant others, we have made an effort to examine some of the factors leading to the burnout syndrome in nurses. Suggestions are made about the ways in which the organizational structure should support nurses who work within that structure. More important, emphasis is placed on nurses' responsibility for seeking and developing their own support systems.

To facilitate its use, we have divided this book into three parts. In Part One, the reader will find an overview of psychoanalytic and attachment theory explanations for the grieving process. Chapter One also includes a section on the use of the nursing process and attachment theory as a framework for planning nursing intervention with the patient who is chronically ill or disabled. Attention is given throughout the book to the fact that family members and significant others (including health professionals) also grieve the losses experienced by a member of their family or client population. A theoretical framework for understanding the sexual health needs and problems of the chronically ill or disabled person is also included in Part One.

Part Two demonstrates the grief responses of individuals to illness from various points on the life continuum and from various perspectives. We have made no attempt to include all major illnesses because to do so would increase the risk of repeating the same conceptual material ad nauseum. Some redundancy does occur across the chapters, but hopefully not to the point of disservice to understanding the important concepts of grief and its resolution. Concepts of crisis intervention are introduced in Chapters Four and Five to indicate other approaches to nursing care.

Part Three focuses primarily on the nurse. Chapter Seven aims to assist the nurse in understanding the phenomenon of hope that is here viewed as the opposite of grief. Considerable effort was made to assist the nurse to examine ways in which she can be instrumental in fostering hope in grieving clients. Chapter Eight recognizes the fact that nurses also respond to stress created by the continued demand to meet the health needs of others. The concept of a hierarchy of needs, as described by Maslow (1954), introduces this chapter and serves as the underlying basis for understanding the burnout syndrome in nurses. However, the notion of a hierarchy of needs applies to patients as well.

It is our hope that the concept of grieving, as it applies to the physically ill or disabled person, is covered broadly enough so that it can be generalized to persons in other illness states even though these are not mentioned by name. The efficacy of any concept lies in the nurse's ability to adapt it to the recipient's specific need. That is, after all, the art of nursing.

Considerable effort was made to avoid the pronouns *he* and *she* in the text. However, since there is no acceptable singular term in the English language that encompasses both genders, these terms were occasionally used in order to avoid awkwardness and distractions in sentence structure. When the word *he* or *she* appears in text the reader should interpret it to mean *he and she*. Certainly no sex bias is intended.

JEAN A. WERNER-BELAND

Acknowledgements

I want to thank my friends and relatives, who shared themselves beyond my greatest expectations in order to help me through my own process of grieving. In addition, I want to thank the fantastic people in nursing, physical therapy, medicine, and occupational therapy who continue to work so hard and so faithfully to help patients regain their optimal functioning, sometimes against almost impossible odds. To those who remember me as "Hospital # 6711," Thank you!

Thanks also to my sister-in-law, Irene, for reading the manuscript and for her many helpful suggestions; to Mildred Gottdank for reading the chapter on hope and to Ellen Jacobsen for her speedy and accurate typing; to all of the contributors and to our editor for their patience with me; and to my husband, Ralph, for being his usual loving, encouraging, supportive, and helpful self.

J W-B

Grief Responses to Long-Term Illness and Disability

PART ONE

Part One focuses on the important theoretical concepts for dealing with the grief responses of the chronically ill or disabled person, his family, and his significant others. The term *significant others* is meant here to include caregivers—doctors, nurses, and others—who are in a position to impact upon the entire being of the person(s) who seeks their help.

Chapter 1, "Theoretical Concepts of Grieving," approaches an understanding of grieving first from the psychoanalytic and then from the attachment theory position. Examples of the use of attachment theory in conjunction with the nursing process in the care of one physically disabled and one chronically ill individual are given.

Chapter 2, "Physical Disability and Grief Resolution," looks at grieving as it occurs in the individual who has acquired a physical disability in late adolescence or adulthood. Some of the external and internal factors that impinge upon the individual and serve as a source for understanding the behavioral reactions of the sick or disabled are discussed.

Chapter 3, "Effects of Grief, Associated with Chronic Illness and Disability, on Sexuality," explores illness-related grief and its effect on sexual identity and attachment, sex role behav-

1

iors, and sexual expression. Guidelines are included for use of the nursing process in relation to the sexual health of the chronically ill or disabled person.

CHAPTER ONE

Theoretical Concepts
of Grieving

Jean A. Werner-Beland

INTRODUCTION

Grief, bereavement, mourning, and other related concepts have recently come to the foreground of our attention with the current interest in death and dying. However, these terms and their meanings should be equally of interest to nurses and other health professionals who work with individuals who have long-term illnesses or acquired disabilities. Although it is assumed that any illness produces some degree of personal disequilibrium, often akin to the grief response, this type of response takes on even greater significance with those individuals who continue to live under less than ideal physical conditions for extended periods. In this latter instance the reference is to those persons whose physical condition is a constant reminder to themselves, and often to others, of the tenuousness of perfect health, or of life itself.

Being thus reminded creates a state of chronic grieving not unlike grief reactions that occur following the loss of a significant other. And yet, in my opinion, the chronic grief response of the ill and/or disabled is unlike that which occurs

3

when the loss is an object outside of oneself. For the chronically ill or disabled individual there is no immediate end to the situation that produces the grief—there is no foreseeable closure or resolution.

When comparing the loss of close family members with the loss of one's body functions, I have found that, for me, the loss of one's own function is quantitatively and qualitatively different from the loss of someone outside of one's self. The grief that is the result of loss of self is unique. When a loved one dies there is hope of resolution of grief. That person is gone and one can learn to live without him. More important, he is not reappearing constantly to reactivate the feelings of loss. On the other hand, the loss of one's own functioning is always present. Although the feelings about this loss also diminish over time, events frequently occur that remind the person that he is less than perfect. Grief raises its ugly head each time the illness or disability becomes conspicuous or when it significantly interferes with hoped-for goal achievement.

Most of what we are able to infer about grief responses to illness or disability derives from knowledge gained from studies of the grief responses of the terminally ill or the bereaved survivor. Kubler-Ross (1969) tells us that once confronted by the knowledge of one's own terminal illness a person essentially goes through five reactive phases: denial and isolation, anger, bargaining, depression, and acceptance. Those who write about the response called depression tend to equate it with grief and anxiety (Jacobson, 1971; Szasz, 1961), although one does see, upon careful reading, that there is an attempt on the part of these authors to differentiate pathological from "normal" depression.

Our lack of data about grief responses to chronic illness and disability make the inferential approach the best that we have at the moment. There is no doubt that the entire area of grief in the chronically ill or disabled needs considerable study.

By way of example, there is some personal documentation in literature that sheds light on the reactions of people who have suffered life-threatening events; reactions that seem to include all of the components of grief as described in the literature. Lair (Lair and Lair, 1973) describes his immediate reaction to having a myocardial infarct as one of "deep calm." He remembers thinking, "I'm never again going to do anything I don't believe in." That decision, Lair relates, helped him through the days immediately following his heart attack—days that he characterizes as oblivion. After being moved from the coronary care unit to a semi-private room, Lair describes himself as playing sick games to keep from thinking about his problems. These games seemed to serve both the purpose of denial and as a vehicle for the expression of his anger. Bargaining for Lair seemed to take on the form of talking to God about wanting to live long enough to see his children grow up (pp. 15–25).

Lair's wife, on the other hand, describes her reaction to this sudden onset of illness in her husband in the more classic terms used by Lindemann (1965), Kubler-Ross, and others. Jackie Lair's disbelief and denial are almost textbook in character. First she describes experiencing waves of physical feeling. Soon thereafter she experienced feeling angry at hospital personnel for controlling her life. Later, in her husband's posthospital readjustment period, it is interesting to note that Mrs. Lair becomes anxious, depressed, and requires psychiatric care. In Lair's early readjustment period he consistently shifted his obsessions from one object to another in rapid succession. It was this behavior that made his family's position more difficult. The reactions of the children are described as being more similar to the reaction of the mother than to that of the father (pp. 31–112).

Jill Kinmont (Valens, 1975) describes her immediate reaction to a skiing accident that resulted in her becoming a quadriplegic, as "Oh, my God, what have I done?" A short time later in the emergency room she feared that she might die. A few weeks after the accident she became aware of the fact that she and her friends were trying to find excuses for what had happened to her (125-36). Throughout this story one sees that the reactions of Jill and her family follow the grieving phases described by Kubler-Ross. The phases, however, seem to take much longer to develop and work through than those described as "usual" where the loss is the death of a significant other. In the case of Jill Kinmont, as well as with others with acquired disabilities whom I have observed, the phases of the grief process seem to evolve in correspondence with each new phase of recovery and rehabilitation. It is interesting to note that Kinmont (Network Television Program, "Tragedy to Triumph," August 29, 1977), in response to a child's question about how it felt not to be able to walk, said that she hadn't walked for twenty years (her accident occurred in 1955) and that she does not think much about not being able to walk anymore. Her response indicates, therefore, that she probably felt different about walking at this point in her life than any of the children would if they suddenly became unable to walk.

Having been injured in an automobile accident that resulted in my receiving some cervical cord damage, I can concur that my immediate reaction to injury was similar to that described by Lair. I remember regaining consciousness while still inside of the car. I knew immediately that my neck was broken. I do not know how I knew that, but I did. A man told me to lie very still because I was badly hurt and that an ambulance was on its way. I remember thinking that he was silly for telling me that I was badly hurt. Couldn't he see that I knew that already? It was not until I was subjected to the various pressures and procedures in the emergency room that I actually felt fear for my survival.

In order to develop further this theme of grief responses, I will discuss briefly some of the psychoanalytic theory that has been forwarded in an attempt to increase the understanding of reactions to loss. Second, I will examine grief responses more fully using concepts from attachment theory. While not casting out the concepts of psychoanalytic theories, I find attachment theory is more compatible with my thinking that grieving is a necessary concomitant of illness or acquired disability, and, therefore, is one part of the loss-adaptation cycle. Third, I will present two case examples of application of attachment theory and the nursing process to the grieving process as it affects the individual, his family, and his caregivers.

OVERVIEW OF GRIEVING

Most people agree that some form of grief reaction follows any loss that to them is significant. Following the loss there is a state of thinking, feeling, and activity that is the direct consequence of the loss of the loved or valued object (Shoenberg, et al., 1970, pp. 20–21).[1] Disagreement arises because of the positions taken by various theoreticians to explain the dynamics of these thinking, feeling, and activity states. Con-

---

[1] For example, a dear old cat that I had for 15 years had to be put to sleep the day I wrote this. The following is a description of my reaction as I recorded it that same day.

I have been crying, angry, and working like a mad woman all afternoon. If I try to attend to the problems of others, then I am O.K. If I am not doing that, my mind wanders and I start crying again. The tomcat is walking around crying and searching and wondering where his mate is. I had to put him in the laundry room for now because seeing him search makes me so sad that I will cry again and I have someone coming for a supervisory session in ten minutes. I wish he had called to cancel the appointment! How am I to attend to his needs when I have problems of my own? Why didn't I call him and cancel? Probably because it will be a distraction, and I need a distraction right now. The muscles in my jaw hurt from keeping them tight so I won't cry. Oh damn! She was only a cat, but I loved her. She was so snooty and discriminating. I remember the day she was born. I picked her out of the litter right away, and then waited until she was weaned so I could take her home. I remember, too, when she had her babies. I kept one so she would have company. She mourned when he was lost. Then a friend gave me another kitten as a replacement. That is Et Tu. Et Tu is mourning and so am I. Goodby dear Armi.

fusion also arises in the use of terms to describe these reactions. However, there is considerable agreement that grief reactions can vary in time of occurrence and in magnitude.

It is possible to experience grief before the actual loss occurs. This is referred to as *anticipatory* grief. Such responses are seen during the terminal phase of a loved one's illness, when a person is witnessing the decline of his own health, when facing the prospect of surgery, when preparing for a child to leave home, and so on. In anticipatory grief many of the behaviors are the same as those which are observable after a loss has occurred. In any event, the anticipatory grief response usually follows the pattern described by Kubler-Ross. In some rare instances it is possible that a person may engage in adaptive behaviors that successfully deny the loss and thus avoid the actual experience of grief, but such instances seem to be rare (Shoenberg et al., p. 27).

THE PSYCHOANALYTIC VIEW OF GRIEVING

Writers having a psychoanalytic orientation concur that grief is a state that occurs after the experience of a significant loss. However, these same writers are also inclined to view grief as maladaptive. In the psychoanalytic view, bereavement, with its accompanying thinking, feeling, and acting states, is equated with illness. The person who experiences grief in conjunction with a significant loss is seen as engaging in behavior that departs significantly enough from the person's usual emotional state to be deemed sick. Thus, in the psychoanalytic view, grief is pathological and should be treated as a disease condition (Shoenberg et al., pp. 20–21).

Brenner (1976) in a discussion of superego analysis, gives an illustration of a young woman in her thirties whose mother was terminally ill with cancer and subsequently died. Although the young woman had spent many hours at her mother's bedside, she was not present when her mother died.

Brenner describes the young woman's guilt and remorse as stemming from ambivalence toward her mother which the young woman had held since childhood. Her response after her mother's death was explained in terms of defenses that were not adequate to avoid guilt and self-reproach for these old feelings (pp. 80–81). Whereas Janet Lair describes feeling angry at nurses and doctors for exercising control over her life, Brenner states that this type of reaction is actually a projection of guilt onto nurses and doctors in order to diminish one's own guilt feelings held in relation to the significant other who becomes ill (p. 81). Although the psychoanalytic view may have validity, it is not beyond the realm of possible reality that someone could legitimately be angry with nurses and doctors for controlling her life.

If we accept the psychoanalytic view as valid, we then view grief responses as manifestations of psychic conflict in relation to danger. This danger may be real or anticipated, but it is especially related to reactivation of feelings stemming from perceived dangers that occurred in the first years of life such as loss of object, loss of love, fear of castration, and superego condemnation, or any combination of these (Brenner, p. 98). When one starts with the premise that loss equals danger, then the situation can be presented schematically as:

DANGER $\longrightarrow$ ANXIETY $\longrightarrow$ SYMPTOM FORMATION

Symptom formation in this instance is variously called grief, bereavement, mourning, depression, or depressive affect, depending on your source.

Brenner contends that in relation to loss:

> The entire range of psychic phenomena that are included under the headings of remorse, penance, propitiation, and even undoing are more apt to be used defensively in connection with the conviction that calamity has occurred than in connection with the sense that one is impending (p. 103).

Brenner also indicates that the foregoing is a general rule and acknowledges that exceptions do occur. Certainly anticipatory grieving, which was referred to previously, must be one exception to this general rule.

Aggression is another frequently observed response to a calamity or loss. Brenner notes that aggression is not without consequence, however. Frequently, the expression of angry or aggressive feelings gives rise to new problems (p. 104). For example, the patient who expresses angry feelings toward the nurse following the amputation of his leg may be conscious to a degree that his feelings are really misdirected. This slight awareness of the fact that feelings are being displaced or misdirected can produce increased psychic discomfort in the patient because he knows he is missing the appropriate object for his aggression. Taking out his aggression on a nurse who has done nothing to merit these feelings may increase the patient's feelings of guilt and may also increase his fear of retaliation. On the other hand, the patient may not know who or what the appropriate object is.

I can remember when I was on a stryker frame, early in the course of my disability, that I was so angry at what had happened to me that I wanted to scream at anyone and everyone who had the courage to enter my room. I knew this was neither appropriate nor would the open expression of such anger be apt to gain me the kind of nursing care I knew I needed. The anger was at times such an intense feeling that even the slightest hint of error on the part of a nurse or doctor seemed to justify my expressions of displeasure. Rightly or wrongly, when the nurse dropped me off of the stryker frame onto the floor, and let me lie there, I perceived this as retaliation for all of my crabbiness. Thinking then that the nursing staff and others were not safe targets for my anger, I became very angry at God. After all, I could tell myself that God must have abandoned me—otherwise why would I be in such a mess! Furthermore, I had dozens of get well cards from well-intentioned people who had written that my accident was "God's will." So, if the condition I was in was "God's will," then God and I were at war. He became a handy target for every angry, miserable feeling I was having.

From a psychoanalytic perspective, my response, I am sure, would have some meaning stemming from unresolved childhood conflicts. From a personal point of view, I am more inclined to say that the anger was a natural consequence of the hopelessness and helplessness I felt at that time. There I was, a quadriplegic, and that is not much when one suddenly feels that a diagnosis is her only distinction. What I had been was gone. At that moment it seemed as if nothing was possible. I could not even have a bowel movement on terms over which I had some control. Do you know what it feels like to lose control over one of the first functions over which one gains mastery in life? True, you learn to walk before you learn to go to the toilet in the proper place at the proper time, but for me walking does not carry with it all of the positive and negative social values that control over bowel and bladder function does. The very act of messing the sheets because of involuntary bowel activity, or, its reverse of having to have one enema after the other to be rid of the stuff was almost more than I could cope with. Nurses would say things like, "I don't know why you are so upset. It's just an enema." I wanted to scream, "I have crapped on my own for 36 years! You just don't understand! I am dead! Some part of me had the audacity to stay alive, but, for the most part, I AM DEAD!!!"

My point is this: Which is more important for the nurse to understand—the psychodynamics of my response as it related to my childhood and early toilet training, or, the meaning that the entire situation was having for me right then and there? Perhaps as a way of answering this we can refer to the writings of Szasz (1961) who does not deny the analytic stance taken by Brenner, but puts object loss and its subsequent reactions into the framework of a game model. Szasz suggests that people do not do well in situations lacking in norms. According to Szasz, people need familiar human objects, and, in addition, they also need familiar norms and rules. Therefore, it can be inferred that without familiar norms, rules, and object relationships, anxiety increases and atypical responses are apt to follow. What could be greater in terms of object loss than the loss of the familiar self, accompanied by the loss of familiar surroundings and activities? Using Szasz' game concept, suddenly there are no known games to play either in the personal or interpersonal spheres. It is, according to Szasz, "necessary to consider the relationships of the ego or self to games. Otherwise one is forced to reduce all manner of personal suffering to considerations of object relationships" (p. 283). What this means to me is that in order to understand a person's response to loss it is vital to look at the internal or intrapsychic meaning of loss to the person, as well as the external or interpersonal meaning. One or the other, and of and by itself, it not sufficient for understanding the responses that loss of function brings about.

According to Szasz, people can suffer considerable loss to life games they consider worth playing without suffering object loss (*object* meaning here those outside of self) (p. 283). There is a striking example of this in a book entitled *You Get Used to a Place* (Randal, 1973). One of the patients in a state mental hospital is a woman who became acutely depressed following a radical mastectomy. Her initial response to surgery had been within normal limits. It was after her husband exhibited shock at seeing the operative site for the first time that she became anxious and felt very much unloved and unwanted. None of this was actually true except for the part about her husband expressing shock at seeing her naked for the first time after surgery. A large measure of his shock was because he felt hurt by the ugliness of her scar and because of what had happened to her, and not because he no longer loved her or thought her to be repulsive. However, she felt so unlovable and repulsive herself that this was how she interpreted his response. She continued to dwell upon this incident while cutting off any attempt by her husband to talk about it. She withdrew from her usual life games to such an extent that she finally required hospitalization (pp. 188–200).

A psychoanalytic interpretation of this case might hypothesize that this woman had always had problems with her sexual identity and that the breast amputation may have been a symbolic castration. All of this could be true, but in order to understand the patient's response, one must understand how she interpreted the loss to herself, as well as how this perception or interpretation became projected onto her significant relationships with her family. Her attentive, not to mention bewildered, husband was still there. Her children were still there. They continued to live in the same house, and they loved her as they always had, but she was no longer able to perceive the old game plans and enjoy them in the same old ways. The result was a problem of such serious proportion that outside help and guidance was required in order to bring it to resolution.

On the other hand, a person may suffer what we perceive to be a serious loss without any significant alteration in game plan. In our society we assume automatically that the loss of a parent is a serious matter. But suppose an offspring has had a life of his own away from this parent for years. The death of the parent may bring about feelings of sadness in the surviving offspring. However, since the relationship was not personally close in terms of day-to-day living, the loss does not seriously affect the offspring's game plan or life style. After a short period of feeling saddened, the familiar norms, routines, and goals are engaged in once more by the offspring. In such a case we would be in error to expect a marked or prolonged grief reaction.

The same reasoning can be applied to the loss of one's body functions. Although a person can be expected to mourn the loss of body functions to some degree, one might expect that the greater the significance of the part and its functions to the person, the greater the reaction when that function is lost. The loss of a leg may be mourned more deeply by the professional athlete than by a man who earns his living sitting at a desk, but this is an assumption and cannot be taken for granted. In evaluating the meaning and significance of a physical illness or disability, the nurse should take into account the intrapsychic meaning of the loss, the interpersonal meaning, the socioeconomic meaning, and so on. Nursing intervention can then derive from an assessment of data obtained from these various dimensions of the patient's life, rather than focusing upon a single and overly simplistic source of information.

A point we frequently forget is that the illness or disability also has avocational as well as vocational meaning for the patient. As nurses we are often remiss because we do not look at the meanings that avocations have for people—meanings sometimes more important than their primary jobs. If the illness or loss does not affect the person's job we tend to minimize its significance. However, how the illness or loss affects one's self-image in terms of total life style is of paramount importance. I think I am an example of this point. I have the rather typical limitations in hand functioning of most quadriplegics (contractures and loss of fine finger movements). This does not affect my work as a psychiatric nurse educator to any great extent. In spite of this functional impairment I can hold a pen and I can write. I can type with two fingers better than some people can with ten. If my students are uncomfortable because they have a "gimp" for a professor, we can talk about it. The point is, if this was all that anyone looked at he would conclude that this limitation in hand functioning is of minimal importance to me. Not so! I have grieved this limitation more than my limitation in walking; probably because events so often bring it into my awareness. If a button comes off a blouse there is nothing I can do about it because I cannot hold a needle to sew it on again. Those kinds of fine finger movements are gone. I used to sew many of my own clothes, but not any more. When I go to church I am supposed to shake hands with those around me as a sign of peace. Did you ever offer a quadriplegic "claw" to someone and watch the expression on his face as he withdraws his hand or hesitates to follow through with his handshake? After a while one gets conditioned to this response, but not entirely.

Hands have always been important to me as a source of expression and creativity. I grew up in an environment where it indeed was accepted as fact that "idle hands are the devil's playthings." Hands are also very practical things that everyone uses every day in more ways than we are even conscious of when they function well. We tend to take hands for granted. It is really practically and psychologically difficult not to be able to button buttons without some kind of an implement, not to be able to zip zippers, or not to be able to knit a sweater or crochet an afghan. Thank God for one thing—after some practice I can still pop tops on beer cans!

What this illustrates is that a person can experience loss through illness or disability at the so-called real or external level and also at the internal or fantasy level (Szasz, p. 284). The significance at either level to one's game-playing strategies in life needs to be recognized if the resolution of grief, which requires the learning of new games, is to be effective. Problems arise when one continues to try to use the same life games without the capacity to do so, or gives up on games in hopeless despair when it is not necessary to do so.

ATTACHMENT THEORY: AN APPROACH TO UNDERSTANDING GRIEF

Bowlby, the major proponent of attachment theory (1960; 1973), views grief as an adaptational response to the loss of an attachment object. Unlike many psychoanalytic theorists, Bowlby takes a holistic approach to the understanding of grief. That is, he looks at the whole object that is lost as being significant and does not subscribe to the part-loss theories of Klein and others. Therefore, the symbolic meaning of parts such as breast, arm, and so forth, gives way to understanding the significance of the lost object in its entirety (Bowlby, 1969, pp. 367-69; Mendelson, 1974, pp. 112-14). This seems to me to be a far more positive approach than one that views all grief as maladaptive or tends to look at loss only in terms of the significance of specific body components. The attachment theory approach also seems to have potential as an aid in defining the roles of helping persons who interact with the grieving ill or disabled person. Although Bowlby studied the reactions of children to temporary or permanent separation from parents (especially the mother) his work seems to have relevance to adults who have sustained losses through chronic illness or physical disability.

Bowlby uses the word *mourning* to refer to the entire series of behavioral and psychological consequences that stem from the loss of a loved object. These processes may take healthy or pathological courses. In Bowlby's terminology, *grief* denotes the sequence of subjective experiences that occur as a concomitant of mourning. *Depression,* for Bowlby, is an aspect of grief that is characterized by "inertia, purposelessness and helplessness and may be seen by the observer as sad, curtailed or disorganized behavior." This use of the term *depression* is distinguished from depressive illness or melancholia. The latter condition (depressive illness or melancholia) is viewed by Bowlby as a clinical syndrome that is pathological (Mendelson, p. 113).

Attachment theory stresses that a person can be expected to operate effectively only in his environment of adaptedness. When the biological structure of the human system is under consideration, then the environment within which this human system is to operate also must be considered simultaneously (Bowlby, 1969, p. 50). For Bowlby the process of becoming adapted can refer to either of two distinct kinds of change:

> First, a structure can be changed so that it continues to attain the same outcome but in a different environment. Secondly, a structure can be changed so that it attains a different outcome in the same or a similar environment (p. 51).

An example of the first kind of adaptation is seen in the Indians of the Andes Mountains. The circulatory and respiratory systems of these Indians have adapted over time so that they now function effectively in the rarified atmosphere in which they live. An example of the second kind of adaptation might be the ill or disabled person who successfully engages in a rehabilitation program and learns to adapt procedures so that he can perform activities of daily living in his usual environment in spite of physical limitations.

It is fortunate that man is versatile and has a great capacity for innovation and change since his environment of adaptedness does not remain fixed or stable for long. External and internal events are continually taking place that alter the environment and require new orientations of self to reestablish maximum effectiveness. In this regard we must concern ourselves not only with an external environment that becomes unstable, but also with changes within the person that are brought about by illness or injury. These changes dictate how the person will relate to his total environment.

Another important concept in attachment theory is that man is more than a goal-directed being. He is, in Bowlby's terms, goal corrected. This means that man's behavior is controlled by systems that are constantly being corrected in reference to discrepancies that exist between current performance and set-goals. Bowlby writes:

> Two vital components of a goal corrected system are: (a) a means of receiving and storing information regard-

ing the set-goal, and (b) a means of comparing the effects of performance with instruction and changing performance to fit (1969, p. 70).

How instructions come to exist within the person is determined, for the most part, by his genetic environment, the epigenetic processes, and those processes called *learning*. Bowlby uses the Tomanian notion of cognitive maps to describe how man finds his way from one part of his familiar environment to another. When deviations of great magnitude occur, and the person has no cognitive map or set of instructions for readily establishing goal-corrected behavior, major disruptions in personal equilibrium also occur. Someone who suddenly becomes physically disabled or blind, for example, must immediately begin to make different plans from those he had when he was physically fit or sighted. Bowlby suggests that such changes in plans for living are usually completed slowly; then they are done imperfectly, and sometimes not at all (1969, pp. 80–82).

Examples of the inflexibility of individuals at a very basic level can be inferred from reports of the content of dreams of persons who became handicapped as adults. Even though these same people are able to make overt adaptive responses to living over time, many report that they never dream of themselves as having any physical problems. Just to name two, I have never dreamed of myself as using crutches even though it is ten years since I first acquired them; my husband does not dream of himself in a wheelchair even though it has been a necessary mode of mobility for him for more than twenty-five years. I suppose a psychoanalyst might say that this omission represents the wish dimension of dreaming. That certainly is possible, since it seems unlikely that any person with a relatively intact ego would actively wish to include a wheelchair or crutches as part of his self-image. The main purpose for including these examples, however, is to illustrate how a person can accept body changes and adapt life functions. He can correct goals (Bowlby) or change game plans (Szasz) and live quite a full life with his given limitations while unconsciously retaining a core of unrelenting adherence to a previous, more preferred, identity.

Where do concepts of attachment and attachment behavior fit into ideas about behavior schemes or goal-corrected behavior? Attachment behavior is defined as seeking to maintain proximity to another individual (Bowlby, 1969, p. 194). It is a type of behavior that develops as an infant matures and it increases until about three years of age. Characteristically, "attachment behavior" encompasses those behaviors that are aimed at keeping another person close, or at returning a person to a proximal position if he leaves. Young children cry, they search, they cling, or they run to the parent. Each of these behaviors is aimed at bringing the attachment object (parent) closer, especially when the child feels alone or afraid. In the adult, attachment behavior is a straightforward continuation of the attachment behavior seen in children.

> In sickness or calamity, adults often become demanding of others; in conditions of sudden danger or disaster a person will almost certainly seek proximity to another known and trusted person (Bowlby, 1969, p. 207).

Or, as is shown in Schacter's fear-affiliation experiments (Jones and Gerard, 1967), where there is no known and trusted person available, an experimental subject in a high fear condition will seek affiliation with strangers who are about to undergo the same experience (pp. 371–72).

While psychoanalytic theory refers to these same behaviors as regressive, attachment theorists view the increase in attachment behavior as a natural consequence of sudden shifts in one's environment of adaptedness. In this sense, attachment behavior plays a vital role in each person's life from the cradle to the grave (Bowlby, 1969, p. 208).

Two forms of attachment behavior have been noted. The first is signaling behavior—that class of behaviors whose aim is to bring the attachment object closer to the person doing the signaling. The second form is approach behavior—that category of behaviors which brings the person closer to the attachment object. Each of these forms of attachment behavior can vary in intensity. As the intensity of the motivating force rises, there is an increase in the number of and variations in the forms of attachment behavior that are observable. It may also be that the less secure the person is and the less sure he is of his relationship with the attachment object, the more he will show strong evidence of attachment behaviors. However, other things need to be considered in the evaluation, such as: (1) the whereabouts of the attachment object; (2) the presence of other persons who are threatening or nonthreatening; (3) the nature of the nonhuman situation; and (4) the condition of the person per se (Bowlby, 1969, pp. 244-50). In the human being, anxiety and distress, along with the companion feelings of anger and guilt, have as their principal source separations or threatened separations from loved figures (attachment objects).

Oftentimes the nature of the stimuli or the objects that frighten us bear only an indirect relationship to what in fact is dangerous (Bowlby, 1973, p. 79). This is an important point to remember when trying to understand reactions to loss or injury. It is not always easy to understand these responses, especially if we look for a one-to-one correspondence between the nature of the person's physical condition and the intensity of his behavioral response. Another point to remember is that we are frightened not only by the presence, or the expected presence, of certain types of situations, but also by the absence, or expected absence, of others. A hospitalized patient, for example, is frequently confronted with both of these states. Perhaps he fears hypodermic injections and knows he is to receive an injection soon. His fear increases because of what is expected. On the other hand, the patient may also become frightened because his usual cues for behavior are absent and he does not know what to expect.

Attachment theory also holds that compound stimuli produce more fear than any single stimulus situation operating alone (Bowlby, 1973, pp. 118–23). Becoming ill or injured, especially when hospitalization is necessary, is a compound stimulus situation. It would be difficult enough to adjust to illness as an isolated event but this is almost never the case. The illness or disability produces a threat to self both in terms of threat to body image and also threat to one's very existence. As a result there is a threat to established relationships; there is the threat that comes from the strangeness of the hospital situation; there is the threat brought on by the absence of usual attachment figures; plus the guilt and anger produced by the presence of the illness with its accompanying fear of retaliation. According to Bowlby, probably nothing increases the likelihood that fear will be aroused more than finding oneself alone in a strange place (1973, p. 118). This, in turn, produces an increase in signaling and approach behaviors. As difficult as it may be for us to accept, not all signaling or approach behaviors are of a congenial sort. For the patient who is grieving the loss of self as the result of illness or disability, signaling and approach behaviors can be so mixed with angry and aggressive behaviors that they become almost one and the same thing. For example, if a person has lost part of his body (i.e., part of his favorite attachment figure—himself), it seems likely that his behaviors, whatever these may be, would be seeking reassurance that (1) he has done nothing bad and is still acceptable to other attachment figures, and (2) no harm will come to him in the form of additional physical and psychological pain.

In order to understand the meaning of the grief responses to illness or disability it is important to view these responses within the context of the person's total environment. The responses can then be seen to be ways that the person uses to gain information and to reevaluate what his many relationships are and will be. If we assume that illness, disability, or any threat to wellness (either current or future), is viewed as a dangerous situation, then we can better understand individual patient's responses. We must keep in mind that what is real danger for one person may not be real danger for you or for me. Therefore, the nurse who evaluates the patient's situation needs to understand where the patient is coming from in terms of the following: (1) the natural clues to danger that he uses (such as strangeness, rapid approach, being left alone), these are fairly universal with all people; (2) the imitative or culturally determined clues to danger that he uses (included here are a whole gamut of "taught" anxieties); and (3) the clues he has gained from other experiences and has added to his repertoire as a means of assessing danger (Bowlby, 1973, pp. 153–61). An example of this third type of clue is the person who, once bitten by a dog, continues to feel afraid around strange dogs.

As mentioned previously, anger is often seen as another response to separation or loss. Bowlby indicates that whenever loss is permanent, angry and aggressive behaviors often occur, but in these situations these behaviors are without function. That is, the angry behavior will not serve to bring back what is lost, although that is the intent. An unwanted, although frequently occurring, side effect of angry, aggressive behavior is that instead of bringing potential attachment figures closer to the person who has suffered the loss, the behavior serves to alienate others and drive them away. In such instances the angry, aggressive behavior crosses the narrow boundary between being a deterrent to further loss and being revengeful (1973, pp. 247–49). Patients who have suffered a loss frequently sound selfish and unfeeling. Their anger may seem irrational and misdirected. However, when the behavior is analyzed within the framework of attachment theory it becomes understandable.

One reason why dysfunctional anger so often accompanies physical illness or disability is because the person usually does not believe, at first, that the loss is permanent. The patient (and others) may act as if it is still possible to recover the lost function, part, or general good health. Not only does the patient act as if it is possible to recover the function or to return to a preillness state, but hidden in this is the notion that this entire situation is reproachable. The person who is in the early phase of a long-term illness or acquired disability frequently is questioning his own worth. He wants people to be close and to reassure him that they still like him and need him even if he is sick or disabled. But the anger, whose aim is to signal the lost part or function to return, works against the formation or continuation of essential human relationships. A frequent target for the patient's anger is doctors and nurses, not only because they are at hand, but also because they are perceived as people who helped to create the loss.

In attachment theory the issue of inner-directedness of attachment is not clearly dealt with. Bowlby writes that attachment behaviors reach their peak at about age three. After that these behaviors become less evident except during periods of stress associated with real or threatened loss. It is my contention that during the process of maturation much of the attachment process becomes inner-directed. That is, an important attachment object in adult life is one's self. Under the stress of illness or suddenly acquired disability, the person loses sight of himself as a trustworthy attachment object. For this and other reasons, which were mentioned previously, attachment behaviors (signaling and approach) become more evident to the nurse and others who have contact with a person who is ill. It is a commonly held belief that when one must reaffirm the worth of self this reaffirmation is accomplished through a process of validating oneself with others. At times the process referred to as "validation of self" is made extremely complex by the person who is seeking reassurance and renewed validation. A case in point is a patient who became anxious and depressed when she had to have an ovarian cyst removed. She had always viewed herself as an invincible object, and even this degree of illness caused her to lose faith in herself and in her ability to control her own destiny. Up until this time in her life she had never felt that her control over situations had been seriously challenged. The nurses and others who took care of her were very puzzled by the intensity of her reactions. Everyone, except the patient, judged that she had undergone a relatively simple surgical procedure. The professional staff had difficulty understanding the patient's anger at her husband and children, her mood swings, her bids for attention while verbalizing her independence, and her angry lashing out at anyone who tried to help her. In this case the patient was referred to a psychotherapy group where she spent many months before reconciling her problems.

It is understandable that problems occur when the quality of anger associated with loss crosses the line of reason and becomes irrational as it did with the woman in the previous example. The person who becomes the target for the expression of this kind of anger often feels helpless and may counterattack. Or, worse yet, relatives and others may simply withdraw; thus leaving the patient feeling less worthy than before, and also frightened and abandoned.

In nursing it is important that we attempt to understand patient behaviors, whether these be aggressive or other, and to look for factors that motivate these behaviors so that we can deal with patients in effective, constructive ways.

NURSING IMPLICATIONS

One frequently hears nurse clinicians and nurse educators proclaim that nursing is a holistic art and science. Rogers, in *An Introduction to the Theoretical Basis of Nursing,* holds the view that "man cannot be explained by laws that govern segments of his being" (1970, p. 43). Therefore, it seems appropriate to develop a nursing schema for the person who is grieving the loss of body function from the viewpoint that this person is a total social, psychological, physical, and spiritual being.

How the patient grieves influences and is influenced by those around him—caregivers, family, friends, employers and employment practices, by cultural norms and social mores. Attachment theory includes a consideration of these elements; thus making the understanding of specific signaling and approach behaviors more meaningful. This means that the patient must be viewed in terms of the internal or intrapsychic meaning of the loss as well as in terms of the external or interpersonal meaning of the loss. Using this approach it becomes possible to evaluate behaviors within the context of the person's total environment of adaptedness.

It is important to remember that two factors are involved in the evaluation of behaviors. First, there are the signaling and approach behaviors that do not remain static but change in character and expression along the phases of the grief continuum. That is, they change from the early phase of denial and isolation to the latter phase of acceptance. Second, we must keep in mind that through the expression of grief behaviors the person seeks reassurance that: (1) he had done nothing wrong and is still acceptable to other attachment figures, and (2) no harm will come to him in the form of additional physical or psychological pain. To successfully offer needed reassurance in either of these domains is not always easy; sometimes it is impossible. Because this is so, the use of the nursing process becomes a vital tool in nursing intervention with the grieving ill or disabled person, his family, and his significant others (including nurses and their colleagues). The following case presentations are included as examples of this process. Physical dimensions of care are omitted here for reasons of brevity rather than as an attempt to negate their importance. The relationship of physical care to the total nursing process is of the utmost importance.

Case Illustration I

Our first example is that of a man who received a cervical cord injury as the result of a jump from his garage roof. The man in our example was showing off for his children; claiming that he could fly with an umbrella just like Mary Poppins. Because of his attempted stunt he acquired a cervical fracture and extensive cervical cord damage that resulted in quadriplegia.

Assessment. This man's wife was frightened and concerned for her husband's well-being. In addition, she was furious at him for attempting "such a stupid trick" and thereby depriving their children of an active, physically able father who had been their source of security as well as her own. The husband felt very guilty about his accident, and it was impossible for the nurse, or anyone, to convince him that he had done nothing wrong. His wife's anger also made it difficult to convince him that he was still acceptable to others and especially to his wife, who was an important attachment object for him. Because he brought his physical state upon himself, through his own actions, he could not be assured of protection from additional psychological pain—either through self-castigation or through the unsympathetic attitudes of others. The range of physical care required by this man also made it difficult to assure him that no additional physical pain would come to him.

The wife's feelings interfered with her ability to learn care procedures that she would be required to perform if her husband eventually were to return home. The wife gave evidence of being unable to attend to procedures relating specifically to her husband's bowel and bladder care. She was unable to handle his penis because of her anger and sense of loss stemming from having her sexually active and loving husband transformed, in an instant, into an almost totally dependent being. In the middle of a demonstration by a nurse on the insertion and care of the husband's catheter, the wife ran from the room. She sat on a chair in the hallway where she cried and spilled out her feelings to another patient who just happened to be there. The nurse completed the procedure and left the room, having made no effort to talk to either the husband or wife about what had occurred. After this and other encounters with his wife, the husband began to behave more erratically. Mood swings became a common event. He would vacillate between mild euphoria (at which time he would verbalize that he would soon be back to his old self) and aloof detachment (during which times he would answer when spoken to but without outward demonstration of feeling). During this same period his children were sending various messages about how much they missed their daddy.

An examination of the data collected about the interacting parties in this example can be summarized as follows:

1. The patient had significant guilt feelings due to the nature of events leading up to his injury.
2. His guilt was compounded by the effect his disability was having on his life roles as husband, father, breadwinner, and so forth.
3. His wife was experiencing mixed feelings, the most evident being anger, which she attempted to control in the presence of her husband, but which surfaced on several occasions.
4. The patient's children were communicating that he had let them down by depriving them of their much needed father.
5. The nursing staff were avoiding dealing with issues affecting the patient's external and internal self.
6. The patient's denial and isolation increased as the internal and external stimuli for guilt mounted, and as the evidence of the extent of his physical disability and the amount of care he required became more certain.
7. Both husband and wife had many strengths, not the least

of these was the fact that they loved each other and their children.

8. The husband and wife had mutual concerns, but they had not been able to share these with each other, and there was a critical need for them to be helped to do this.

Planning. The interactional problems identified in this example required at least two levels of action: (1) A planned approach was needed for dealing with the nurses' resistance to intervening in the emotional-interactional component of care; (2) A plan of intervention based upon patient-family needs had to be devised. The nursing diagnosis was that help was needed that would facilitate expression of feelings and the beginning resolution of problems so that physical management instructions could proceed and future-oriented goals could be established.

Goal Identification
1. Identify ways in which unresolved feelings interfere with nursing care and discharge preparation.
2. Establish conferences with husband and wife and nurse to discuss problems.
3. Increase understanding of husband's condition and his responses to it.
4. Explore relationship of identified problems to other needs and concerns. Plan appropriate action.

Implementation
1. Arrange time to meet with husband and wife (and children, if possible).
2. Ask what their concerns are. Recognize with them that the husband has an acquired disability that has imposed changes on their lives.
3. Share some of the nursing observations regarding their

interactions with each other and with staff. Give specific examples.

4. Recognize with the husband and wife (and children, if present) that feelings often seem overwhelming when events such as what has happened to them occur. Suggest that it will be helpful to them and to the nurses in planning care if such feelings are shared.

5. Encourage the setting of short-term realistic goals.

Evaluation. Evaluation implies the collection of additional data in order to determine by means of some preestablished criteria whether or not intervention has a positive, negative, or neutral effect.

In this example it would have done no good to try to convince the husband that he should not feel guilty about the actions leading up to his accident. At the practical level, a nursing goal would be to help him accept the fact that he should stop punishing himself and direct his energies toward more positive goals. Both husband and wife needed to look at the realities of what was still possible for them and the alterations they would need to make in order to maximize their future. They also needed help from the nurse to think about the outside resources available to them and how these resources would help meet some of their needs in order for them to achieve their new goals.

Nursing conferences needed to focus on the attitudes of the caregivers toward the patient and his significant others. Answers were needed to questions such as: What were these attitudes? Where do such attitudes spring from? What values of the caregivers had the patient violated? What values had the wife violated? and so on. The nurses (and other staff) needed to understand that the patient was signaling for help and reassurance through his various behaviors. In some ways he seemed to be clinging to people and wanting to keep them close to him, as if this closeness would help to fill the void created by the real and/or symbolic meanings that the loss had for him.

Many nurses identified that they held rather negative attitudes toward the patient and that these attitudes had been communicated to the patient either verbally or nonverbally. The patient undoubtedly had incorporated his perception of staff attitudes into his response system. Therefore, it is highly probable that these attitudes, as well as those of his wife, affected the way the patient felt about himself. The combination of external forces as well as his own internal perceptions helped to determine the coping patterns that the husband used—namely, denial and isolation. He had not openly grieved his loss, nor had his wife. Both needed to be permitted to do so before there could be any expectation that positive actions would be forthcoming.

Perhaps one of the reasons why divorce is common after one partner becomes disabled is because neither partner received the help that was needed to resolve the grief associated with his or her loss. Each partner becomes preoccupied with the personal meaning that the loss has for him or her. Without outside help they often have increasing difficulty relating to each other in any shared way. One goal of nursing intervention should be to reduce the separation brought on by such self-preoccupation. Specific points in the evaluation of the foregoing case are as follows:

1. Observe husband's and wife's moods during and after discussions.
2. Look for signs of improved ability on the part of the wife to participate in husband's care.
3. Is there, as one would expect, less denial and more open expression of feelings?
4. Is there increased understanding on the part of all persons interacting in this situation?
5. Is there increased willingness to look realistically at the limitations imposed by the injury?

6. Is there increasing evidence of hope and the accompanying ability to engage in realistic plans for the future?

Case Illustration II

Our second example involves a male patient with a progressive disabling disease. The patient and his wife were referred to a psychiatric-mental health clinical nurse specialist by another nurse because they were having "severe disagreements because of their sexual incompatibility."

Assessment. When first seen by the clinical specialist, the two partners stated that they loved each other, but the husband added, with considerable feeling, that at times he wanted to kill his wife because she was an absolute animal when it came to sex. Further exploration revealed that a medication prescribed for the husband was having the side effect of making him sexually impotent. He also was in considerable pain and often felt too sick to perform sexually.

The wife was not sick. She was a normal woman with average sexual needs and needs for socialization. However, she was not aware of the extent of her husband's fatigue and impotence. Instead of talking to her husband about the problem of his sexual abstinence, she had asked her husband's doctor if it was all right for her and her husband to have sexual intercourse. The doctor had answered that whenever they felt like it, it was O.K. The wife had interpreted the doctor's remark to mean "there is no necessity for restriction." When the husband angrily retreated from his wife's sexual advances, she interpreted this as a brutal rejection.

Before he became ill the husband had been the authoritarian master of his household. His wife had always assumed a dependent posture. She liked things the way they had been; as a matter of fact, they both did. They said that they had always had arguments but earlier in their marriage they would resolve their differences by talking things out (somewhat), then they would have intercourse and their angry feelings would be gone. As the husband's illness progressed they talked less and less about the changes in their lives. The wife denied the illness and still clung to old patterns of problem resolution. Therefore, to her, an argument meant that they should talk a little, go to bed and have intercourse, and everything would be all right. The husband had not shared with her the fact that he could no longer perform sexually. Knowing his own physical state, he did not expect to use this old pattern of problem resolution. However, instead of telling his wife this he just expected her to understand what the problems were and to behave accordingly. It also became apparent that as the husband's illness progressed he partially denied the severity of what was happening to him. He also was enraged because he had no control over his life. Remember, this was an authoritarian man who was accustomed to exercising a great deal of self-control, as well as control over his wife and his employees.

Instead of communicating his concerns openly to his wife, his signaling and approach behaviors consisted of making ever greater demands upon his wife's time. He wanted her to stay close (but not too close) and to feed and dress him without making him feel helpless and useless (impotent). These expectations placed his wife in an impossible situation. Without clear communication from him, she constantly misinterpreted his need for closeness. Further, it was impossible for her to do the things for him that his physical condition demanded without his feeling helpless. If she had not dressed him and fed him he would have died naked and starved. On the other hand, when she did these things he became angry at the ignominy of requiring such help and he would vent his anger on her. Certainly this situation had all of the elements of a no win game.

The wife, not knowing what internal meaning all of this was having for her husband, interpreted events according to the internal meaning they held for her. The result was a total breakdown in communication, including many distorted interpretations of the other's intent. By denying the illness the wife desperately tried to avoid confronting the necessity of giving up her dependent role. The husband denied that he was becoming more dependent and having to give up his dominant role. As a couple they had withdrawn more and more from social activities because they were always arguing and could not even agree on who to invite to their home or who to go and visit. The husband stated that he was extremely self-conscious because of his changing physical appearance—another point he had not previously shared with his wife.

In discussion with the nurse clinician it was also revealed that both partners had become very angry at the nurse clinician because she would not assure them that everything would be all right. To them the nurse clinician was "just like the other nurses who had never had one damn thing to say that was good!" This was interpreted to the couple by the nurse clinician as their asking for help to restore control over their lives so everything would be just as it had been before the husband became ill. The nurse said, "I cannot do that. There are circumstances over which none of us has any control. The best we can do is look at alternatives for bettering a bad situation so the two of you can live together with a greater degree of understanding and comfort."

The nursing assessment revealed, in summary, that:

1. This couple did not discuss their problems openly with each other.
2. They were clinging to old coping patterns and because these no longer worked they became frustrated to the point where there was a threatened dissolution of a previously happy marriage.
3. Both were denying the illness and the meaning it had for each of them.

4. Each expressed considerable anger at the other not only as a result of frustration, but, more importantly, as a distancing or isolating maneuver so that neither would have to face the reality of the illness.
5. They were afraid of continued closeness because they did not know what to expect due to changes in the husband's health status.
6. They made unreasonable demands on each other because neither stopped to listen to what the other was saying, if indeed the other sent clear messages at all.
7. Because denial was so strong, neither partner had permitted any evidence of grieving either in self or in the other.

Planning and Implementation. Some planning took place immediately, that is, during the course of talking with the couple. Outside of the actual sessions, short-term and long-term goals were also identified by the nurse clinician. The husband and wife were also asked to state what their goals were in seeking help. They quickly identified that they did not want their marriage to break up, but that they could not go on living the way things were.

A short-term goal was to get them to listen to each other. This was accomplished by telling them directly that they did not listen. When they interrupted each other, the clinician stopped the one doing the interrupting and asked why he or she did not want to hear what the other one was saying. They were encouraged to speak directly to each other and to share their feelings directly instead of telling the nurse clinician. Even though both partners were always present and could hear what was being said, the intent of making them face each other directly was to give them practice in what they were expected to do outside of the sessions. That is, filtering every statement through the nurse clinician had the effect of putting the real intended receiver in the emotional position of receiving messages secondhand. This kind of communication "by-pass" needed to be limited whenever possible.

The long-term goals for this couple consisted of helping them to identify the source of their problems and to alter behaviors to produce more mutually satisfying outcomes. Intervention consisted of direct confrontation in regard to their fears about and denial of the husband's illness. The extent of the husband's physical problems was discussed. For the first time the husband told his wife that he was impotent and that he felt this to be a great threat to his self-image. He also told her that her sexual overtures only magnified his feelings of worthlessness. Because he perceived her as hurting him psychologically, he wanted to hurt her physically. At this point his wife heard what he was saying and understood, to some extent, why he behaved as he did. Thus, with help, the husband's signaling and approach behaviors began to have new meaning for the wife.

Another issue that surfaced, aided by an interpretation from the nurse clinician, was that the wife was angry with her husband for being ill and threatening her security. The husband was angry with his wife for being well. Their attempts to isolate themselves from each other through anger, denial, and actual physical withdrawal were pointed out. They spent considerable time discussing and coming to an understanding of the function that anger served in keeping them apart—even when they were desperately trying in behavioral terms to tell each other that they really wanted and needed to be together.

A second step in intervention was to help this couple define new levels of closeness and to find alternative ways of expressing their love for each other. (Here again, a redefinition of signaling and approach behaviors was needed.) In addition, social activities were discussed at length; taking into account what the husband felt comfortable doing. Together they identified friends and relatives they would be comfortable visiting and other kinds of activities they would consider attending together. They practiced stating clearly what each

wanted the other to hear. Both husband and wife made con-
certed efforts to listen to each other and to ask for clarification when needed instead of operating on private perceptions
and distortions.

It was also identified that both partners tried to bargain
with the nurse clinician and others on the health team. For
example, the husband or wife would say, in effect, "If you
(nurse) will tell me that I (he) am (is) not ill, then I will listen
to what you are saying about our problems." Several times it
was pointed out that bargaining was being used as a means of
reinforcing their denial. The bargaining not only served to
avoid acceptance of the illness, it also delayed the development of a more positive level of adjustment that would
become possible only when both partners were able to face
the reality of what was happening in their lives because of
illness. In addition, the bargaining had a negative effect on
the care they received. Some caregivers, being fully aware
that no bargain was possible, avoided interacting with this
couple because the caregiver was hesitant to say "I cannot
make that kind of bargain with you."

Evaluation. The success of planned intervention was
based upon reports of greater personal comfort and sense of
closeness. Another guideline was the couple's reports of
modifications in the behaviors that had been distressing to
both of them. There was a lessening of the angry outbursts
and threats, and this led to an increase in mutually satisfying
behaviors. Both husband and wife reported that they had
great moments of happiness that came from sitting close
and holding hands, lying close to each other in bed, or from
an occasional spontaneous kiss that carried with it no
demand for further involvement. They also were able to plan
for the future; to accept the husband's prognosis and the
further limitations that time and the progression of his illness
would bring.

When last seen by the nurse clinician, this couple was reporting that they still had occasional arguments, but now each one made more of an effort to stop and to try to talk about what was happening. By no means was a complete state of bliss ever reached, but there were more moments of caring and sharing. These changes were interpreted by the nurse clinician to mean that there was less acting out of feelings associated with grieving and a greater ability to examine and understand these feelings; thereby bringing the grieving process closer to resolution for both parties.

One final consideration in understanding the grief process in illness or disability, and one that I think is illustrated by the previous case example, is that the patient often goes through the phases of grieving at a different rate than do members of his family or his close associates. Nurses who work in rehabilitation settings have told me that they have observed this same phenomenon. Oftentimes the family moves more quickly through the phases of grieving than does the patient. The family members resolve their grieving and are then ready to move on to other goals and activities. The patient, for whom grieving is a longer-term process, does not understand his family's seeming lack of sensitivity to his feelings and needs. The family, not understanding the patient's continued mood swings and grieving behaviors, often becomes impatient. The end result may be a build-up of tension between the patient and other members of his family or his significant others, whoever these may be.

The grief that nurses and other caregivers experience in relation to patients with whom they develop close, caring relationships is an area needing extensive study. I have no doubt that in my role as a nurse I have grieved for many patients. I would like to say that I have grieved with them, but I would not always allow myself that freedom. I suspect the same is true for many health professionals. We experience the feelings and the turmoil of grief in relation to many patients, but we are socialized into professional roles in such a way that we feel it is inappropriate for a professional person to express these feelings. Therefore, we go around with a burden of feelings that we are ashamed to express; even to our colleagues.

As a patient, I sometimes perceived what I thought was the shared grieving on the part of some nurses in relation to me. No one ever said anything to me directly, some just withdrew. I have talked to nurses who, when they thought it safe to do so, would tell me that they experience a wide range of feelings about patients, but that nurses who become patients are especially disturbing to them because the identification potential is so great. A nurse working in a rehabilitation setting recently commented that a nurse who becomes disabled is very threatening to her because, "Then I know I am just as vulnerable as she is. I am not invincible." Chapter 8 attempts to deal with some of the problems facing nurses who care for chronically ill and disabled patients on a day-after-day basis. However, little is known about the effect that a nurse's grief has upon the source of that grief—who also happens to be the recipient of her care.

REFERENCES

Bowlby, J. 1969. *Attachment and loss, volume 1: attachment.* New York: Basic Books, Inc., Publishers.

Bowlby, J. 1973. *Attachment and loss, volume 2: separation, anxiety and anger.* New York: Basic Books, Inc., Publishers.

Brenner, C. 1976. *Psychoanalytic techniques and psychic conflict.* New York: International Universities Press, Inc.

Jacobson, E. 1971. *Depression.* New York: International Universities Press, Inc.

Jones, E. E., and Gerard, H. B. 1967. *Foundations of social psychology.* New York: John Wiley & Sons, Inc.

Kubler-Ross, E. 1969. *On death and dying.* New York: Macmillan Publishing Co., Inc.

Lair, J., and Lair, J. C. 1973. *Hey God, what should I do now?* Greenwich, Conn.: A Fawcett Crest Book.

Lindemann, E. 1965. Symptomatology and management in acute grief. In *Crisis intervention: selected readings,* ed. H. J. Parad. New York: Family Service Association of America.

Mendelson, M. 1974. *Psychoanalytic concepts of depression.* 2nd ed. New York: Spectrum Publications, Inc.

Randal, V. 1973. *You get used to a place.* New York: Berkley Publishing Corporation.

Rogers, M. 1970. *An introduction to the theoretical basis of nursing.* Philadelphia: F. A. Davis Company.

Schoenberg, B.; Carr, A. C.; Peretz, D.; and Kutscher, A.H., eds. 1970. *Loss and grief: psychological management in medical practice.* New York: Columbia University Press.

Szasz, T. S. 1961. *The myth of mental illness.* New York: A Delta Book.

Valens, E. G. 1975. *The other side of the mountain.* New York: Warner Books.

CHAPTER TWO

Physical Disability and Grief Resolution

Jean A. Werner-Beland

INTRODUCTION

Specific problems and issues confront the adult who has an acquired, visible, physical disability. Of importance here are the various factors that affect the individual in terms of grief resolution during the process of resocialization. Many of these factors also apply to individuals with nonvisible disabilities. The distinction between visible and nonvisible disability is not always clear.

Cogswell (1968), in a study dealing with the self-socialization of paraplegics into the community, defines a socialization model as follows:

> A socialization model focuses attention on the processes by which individuals acquire new roles and leads to questions on the development of new self-definitions, skills, activities and associations. Socialization proceeds through interaction among novices (individuals learning new roles) and agents (individuals responsible for training). [p. 11]

41

The acquisition of these new roles and associations, the development of new self-definitions, the learning of new skills and suitable self-satisfying activities are all part of grief resolution, both for the newly disabled and his significant others.

Perhaps one of the major differences between grief associated with long-term illness or disability and grief associated with the loss of a significant other is that in physical illness or disability the person is there to mourn his own loss. While the widow (or widower) can leave her (his) grief and rejoin family and friends in a full range of activities, the disabled person cannot do this. In addition, those closely associated with the newly disabled person mourn his loss because it has significance for them also. Through this interactional process, the newly disabled person not only has his own burden of grief, but he also feels the impact of others' grieving for him and because of him. Resolution of grief in this instance must, by virtue of the fact that the source of the grief is still present, involve all of the principal characters in this life drama. If professional intervention does not involve significant others in the process of rehabilitation and grief resolution, the difficulty of the task will be compounded.

Important questions for both the agents and the novices in such situations are: (1) What new role concepts does the disabled person need to acquire? (2) What significant role modifications does the disabled person and his significant others need to make? (3) What general methods can be employed by which these people will be able to make such changes? and, (4) What social, cultural, economic, and personal factors operate to permit or prohibit these changes from being made? The "how" of learning to make needed changes is especially important since a major dilemma for the newly disabled person falls within the category of remastering social skills and in regaining a sense of social competence. Learning to relate once again to people in the so-called normal world is no small task.

For the professional agent or helping person it may be important to know what attitudes the disabled person and his significant others held toward disability prior to his joining that group. If all were fairly accepting of persons with deviations from physical perfection, they might find it easier to accept disability. Unfortunately, there is little hard evidence to support this assumption. Another important variable is how did this person and his significant others handle crises prior to his becoming disabled? Seligman (1975) tells us that prior immunization to traumatic events, that is, learning to exercise some control over seemingly uncontrollable events, may make it easier for the individual to cope with new traumatic events. From this it should follow, and Seligman's evidence supports this, that the fewer coping mechanisms a person acquires prior to illness or disability, the greater will be his difficulty in dealing with this new crisis (p. 55).

SOCIAL ATTITUDES TOWARD THE DISABLED

Some studies in sociology and psychology give evidence concerning the effects that visible physical disability have on attitudes of the able-bodied person with whom the disabled person must interact (Clore and Jeffery, 1972; Comer and Piliavin, 1972; Davis, 1961; Goffman, 1963; Kleck et al., 1966; Richardson et al., 1961). Goffman (1963) states that in interpersonal interactions the mere presence of a disabled person tends to generate anxiety in the nondisabled person. In response, both individuals quickly become uncomfortable, and the result is often early termination of their interaction. Research subjects in a study by Kleck et al. (1966) were prone to maintain greater physical distance from the disabled confederate than from the confederate who was not playing a disabled role (p. 226). Thus some evidence does exist that confirms the belief that the visibly disabled person serves as a negative stimulus object in individual interpersonal situations.

On the other side of the ledger, Byrne (1961) tells us that studies demonstrate that "once the environmental situation permits or encourages interaction, then affiliation need becomes a helpful variable in predicting individual differences in individual behavior" (p. 713). These are issues of importance because it is not only the disability itself that influences one's responses, but also the effect that the disability has on the quality of interactions with others. Both of these factors influence the disabled person's attempts to resolve his grief and to reestablish a realistic self-definition.

Cogswell (1968), in her study, identified three phases in the resocialization process of paraplegics that pinpoint how the disabled person often approaches the task of achieving a new self-definition. These phases are: (1) severance of many predisability relationships, (2) formation of and testing of new relationships with persons in lower status positions than oneself, and (3) finally moving to reestablish relationships with persons of like status. Cogswell also identified three criteria that the disabled person uses to select settings in which to test out resocialization processes following disability. These are: (1) physical accessibility of the setting, (2) the flexibility and ease with which one can leave the setting, and (3) the conspicuousness of the disability within a particular setting. In these ways the disabled person either consciously or unconsciously maneuvers to maintain or regain his or her integrity (pp. 13–14). The aim is to minimize encounters in which the loss once again becomes evident to the disabled person; thereby reactivating the experience of grief.

For most people who become ill or disabled it takes time for the full impact of what has happened to be fully realized. Isolated messages get through now and then, but it takes considerably longer before all of the implications of the illness or disability actually develop. Just because the body has changed in some way, it is still very difficult to realize that almost everything associated with that person has changed to some degree. In the event of sudden illness or injury, the change occurs with such rapidity that comprehension of its meaning becomes even more difficult for all concerned— patients, relatives, nurses, and others.

In our materialistic society I suppose each of us should have learned that it is the house and not the spirit within, that serves as the initial basis for most value judgments. Becoming disabled is like moving into a new house in a new neighborhood. Shortly after the move one looks out expecting to see the same old familiar sights. It takes time before one can look out with the realization that there is a whole new world out there. For a time the disabled person feels as if he or she has moved into a slum. Because of personal problems with grief resolution and resocialization, as well as with those problems that society imposes on the disabled person, some even lose the desire to go to the window.

The problems of personal adjustment for the disabled person are further complicated by the necessity of having to check on the accessibility of facilities; especially in public places. Should the person forget to check on details of access he may get to his destination only to find steps, revolving doors, or other physical barriers that make it difficult, if not impossible, for him to enter. It is shocking to realize that the unspoken message in many public places says to the disabled person, "You may not enter here!" even when the disabled person desires to be accepted and as self-sufficient as possible.

It is possible then for society, through its interactions with and its reactions to the disabled, to help create a group of *sociogenic neurotics*. This term refers to a group of persons who once adapted in some way within their social environment, but now, because of physical limitations can no longer make old methods of adaptation work for them. Social attitudes and social barriers add to the difficulty of learning new modes of adaptation. This group of disabled persons oftentimes have received little in the way of help that was needed and appropriate to assist them to learn new adaptive patterns. Without this help the person's grief remains unresolved and patterns of flight (withdrawal) or fight (aggression) are often the result.

RESOCIALIZATION, GRIEF, AND DEVIANCE

Three interconnecting issues are critical to understanding why the newly disabled person reacts as he does. These are: *resocialization,* with all of its implications; *deviance,* with its many implications, both personally and interpersonally; and *grief,* with its many facets and nuances. I say these are interconnected because for me it is impossible to separate one's view of self (as this is reinforced by fantasy as well as reality) from how one grieves the loss of limb or function. It is also impossible to separate one's ability to engage in necessary grief work from the process of resocialization. It is impossible to separate the conceptualization of illness or disability as a form of deviant behavior, and the way one reacts to that interpretation of his disability, from the processes of grieving and resocialization. Safilios-Rothschild (1970) states that, "the disabled may react differently to their being labeled 'deviant' and consequently discriminated against." The disabled may move from one to another of many defensive stances, depending upon the reactions of the nondisabled, especially their significant others, to their disability and the postdisability phase of grief resolution and rehabilitation in which they find themselves (pp. 117–118).

Pinpointing the exact moment when one begins grieving his losses after becoming disabled is difficult. For me it began when I was being transferred from a wrecked car to an ambulance. I often think that it was merciful that I kept losing consciousness every few seconds, but even now I can recall that the ambulance signified an emergency and I knew I was it. As a nurse, I had associated emergency with ambulances for many years. I suppose most people are also so conditioned. Not many people are likely to rent an ambulance, crawl on a stretcher, and ride down the highway just for the thrill of hearing the sirens screech or to see the lights flash.

It was not until I was in the emergency room that I actually felt the impact that my condition had on my status as a person. Because I could not sign the admission form, I was threatened with not being admitted for treatment. Because the nursing personnel liked the turtlenecked sweater I was wearing, they pulled it off over my head in spite of my telling them to cut it off because I knew my neck was broken. And, because the doctor had not arrived I was not permitted to lie down even though I asked that I be allowed to do so, all the while insisting that someone have the good sense to stabilize my head and neck.

Confronted with such circumstances one can only feel deviant, although I never would have thought of that label at that time. I was only acutely aware that these people did not have the foggiest notion about how to treat me since I was paralyzed and could not write; neither would they listen to anything I was saying. They only knew how to interact with people who could follow all the rules as these were rigidly defined. Never before had I been so struck by the fact that personnel in hospitals do not know how to adapt procedures and routines to meet the needs of a person who has limitations that involve mobility and motor skills.

Until the moment when I was threatened with not being admitted for treatment, I had not grasped the full impact of what had happened to me. I realized I was in an emergency room, and I knew that my neck was broken, but I had been feeling more like a spectator than the victim. That was short-lived. With the lack of response to my requests, compounded by the demand that I make my paralyzed hands move to sign my name, I experienced a feeling of panic to which I have known no equal. What struck me was the fact that I had no control over anything anymore; not over my own body, not over anyone in the room, and certainly not over what they were going to do to me or with me.

LOSS OF CONTROL AS A CONCOMITANT
OF GRIEVING

It is the awareness of one's inability to control events that produces fear. Seligman (1975) writes that this fear can be useful because it maintains the search for a response that will work to regain control. When there is certainty that the trauma, whatever it may be, is uncontrollable, then fear decreases. It decreases because it is a useless expenditure of energy in a hopeless situation. Once the situation is perceived as hopeless, depression ensues (p. 55).

About five months after I became disabled, a friend and I decided to tape record some of our reactions to my accident. By this time I had regained the ability to walk with the assistance of crutches, but was still a patient in a rehabilitation hospital. The following interchange illustrates Seligman's points as referred to in the previous paragraph:

G: After four or five days in there (intensive care unit) it looked to me like you went through two or three changes in quick succession. One of them was a shocky phase. Then, about the second day, you seemed to realize you were living and so glad to be alive. . . . Shortly after that, like maybe the next day, you were actively wishing you were dead.

J: I remember just before I started crying that I had such a feeling of despair. I can't remember what happened. Something happened and I felt that I was reduced to the lowest, most ignominious point.

G: I know what it was.

J: I was trying to urinate in an emesis basin.

G: That's right. That's been a problem throughout this. That time and another time when you were here (at G's home) and having trouble. It seems that these particular times when you were faced with your own helplessness, about what are ordinarily private bodily functions, that you really despaired.

J: After that I remember I was very quiet. I think because I had to make a decision about whether I was going to live or die. I don't know if it is true that one can make a decision about living or dying, but that was sure the way I felt.

G: You mentioned this before, and also the guy next to you asking if you had made your decision.

J: Yes.

G: Whether to live or die, and telling you that he had made his decision.

J: Yes.

G: Whether it's right or not that you really do have a decision to make, apparently he shared your feeling about it.

J: It was terrible. I thought I had to make this decision between dying, which would be easy, or living and taking a chance on being very crippled and possibly never getting any better. Finally, after a tremendous struggle, I made the decision to live, knowing full well there would be a chance that I'd get some better, or, I'd get no better, or, I'd get a whole lot better.

G: You know, all of this in the intensive care unit fits with my perception of the stages you went through. Right after the despair and wishing to be dead, the next thing you were talking about was trying to adjust to the idea of being a cripple. That's the way it came, in that order.

Notice that implicit throughout this account is the need to control events—even to the point of needing to feel in control of my life or my death. Once this struggle had been surmounted I did not feel as helpless or as despairing as I had previously.

The feeling of helplessness is worse than feeling nothing because, to me, feeling helpless is the ultimate in psychic pain.

During the seven months I spent in hospitals I grew to know the feeling of helplessness very well. Helplessness and I were never on friendly terms, but eventually we became known to each other as two forces struggling for the right of survival. Every time I won a round over helplessness, I felt elated. Every time I lost a round to helplessness, I felt despair. Feelings never were on an even keel in those days. Although I do not think that my behavior was as erratic as were my feelings, others must have observed many of my mood swings. I do not think I am accomplished enough as an actress to hide feelings of such great magnitude.

The point is this: early on as a patient one begins to experience loss. There is much in the literature about the denial of grief, but I think complete denial would take ultrastrong ego defenses because the system of the hospital and of society is a constant reminder of one's deviance and loss. The system determines in great measure when and if the disabled will be allowed to become a person again. The patient is constantly made aware by some personnel (but certainly not all) that he or she is nothing. Fortunately, this attitude is not universal or there would be no resolution of grief and, therefore, no rehabilitation.

Denial obviously functions in the service of allowing the patient to delude himself that he has some control over life events. Not too infrequently someone behaves in a thoughtless manner that jars the newly disabled person out of his denial into the awfulness of reality. I can laugh now about the two elderly volunteers who came into my room one day when I was half-asleep. At the time I was in a face-up position on the stryker frame, and even though I was aware that these women were staring at me I feigned sleep just because I did not have the energy to talk to them. The volunteer who was known to me said to the other one, "Don't you suppose she used to be pretty? It's such a shame!" That opened my eyes both literally and figuratively, and I told both of them to get out of my room and leave me alone. I either cried or experienced waves of empty nausea all the remainder of that day. After all, I had no mirror to see what I looked like. It had not entered my head that I looked bad to other people. I knew I must look somewhat different, since I had tongs sticking out of my head, but since I could not see what I looked like I simply had not dealt with that issue. This experience certainly stripped me of my denial and catapulted me into openly experiencing my grief. Maybe I should thank the old ladies. However, I think there is a better way of helping patients face reality through planned nursing intervention, which, while not without emotional pain, would provide the patient with opportunities to talk about his feelings.

ROLE REDEFINITION AND GRIEVING

Important elements in the disabled person's ability to grieve, cope with his newly acquired deviance, and to emotionally redefine self, derive from family roles, sex roles, social roles, and work roles. Each of these role definitions takes on different degrees of importance at various stages of illness and rehabilitation. I know that I gave fleeting attention to each of these roles while I was still in intensive care, but it was not until later, when I was sure I would live, that I actually began to zero in on what each of these roles meant to me in terms of a "remaining self" and a "lost self." For each individual, and his reference groups, the significance of these roles depends to a considerable extent upon the importance that each held prior to the onset of the disabling condition: at the personal level, at the social systems level, and at the cultural level. The person's predisability life style must be taken into account or it becomes impossible to understand where the disabled person's feelings come from and why he reacts as he does. For the helping person, this approach makes it easier to determine what are the internal as well as the external stimuli which have significance for the disabled person.

D'Affliti and Weitz (1977) imply that grief resolution requires reconciliation of the past with the present. After the initial period of denial it did not seem that any part of the grieving process linked me to my past to give me hope to build on what was possible. Rather, grief in the period that D'Affliti and Weitz refer to as "developing awareness" (p. 141), seemed a state in which all hope had been cut off. The only way to begin again, it seemed, was to get rid of the past and start a new life. It is very improbable that anyone can wipe out years of existence and start as a new being, yet that is what I felt I must do. It seemed that I must destroy all that had been, although this was demonstrated more through behavior than it was thought about consciously.

As soon as I was out of the hospital, I gave away many reminders of my past such as skates, golf clubs, tennis racket, and bike. The interesting part of this activity, as I look back on it now, was that I was very careful to give these items to someone close to me. I knew I could not sell the items even though I could have used the money. I needed to give them to someone who would not take them too far away. At some level of awareness I must have hoped that my old self would live on through the new owner.

C. S. Lewis (1961) describes grief in resolution as a "long valley, a winding valley, where any bend may reveal a totally new landscape" (p. 69). For the person with an acquired disability, the phase of grieving frequently referred to as resolution is not strikingly different from Lewis' description. If and when the disabled person can allow himself to look to new experiences, each of these experiences is like an adventure. I wish I had some magic that would explain just how the transition from grieving and despair to hope and excitement with each new accomplishment takes place—if it takes place. The person who continues to downgrade every achievement and refuses to let the old self die tends to remain unrehabilitated.

D'Affliti and Weitz (1977) write that it is not only the patient, but his family and others who must work through the phases of grieving. While the patient is grieving his loss and trying to understand what that loss means in terms of his many roles, the family also experiences the loss in terms of its meaning to their entire system of role relationships. The family, as a system, needs to understand how its meaningful relationships are affected by this one family member's altered capacity to sustain his previously designated role within the family system. D'Affliti and Weitz give an example of a man who had suffered a stroke and the help he and his wife needed to move past the phase of denial in order to move on toward grief resolution. In this example, the husband often cried because he felt depressed about his body changes, his inability to work, and so forth. At these times his wife became anxious and countered with statements that directed her husband to remain cheerful. In order for resolution to occur, the husband needed help in expressing his feelings and the wife needed help in learning to listen to what her husband was saying (p. 143).

For some individuals, and I feel fortunate to be able to include myself in this group, something happens in the process of grief resolution that allows and even encourages one to find pleasure in many small accomplishments. One such event happened when I was out of the rehabilitation facility only a few weeks. I was living by myself and feeling as if I was just getting by, but not wanting to admit it. One evening one of the faculty members with whom I worked helped me put some nonskid strips in the bathtub, I put down two strips and Elinor did the rest. But at least I managed two without making a total mess of things. More important, she waited to take over at a point when I nonverbally indicated that it was all right for her to do so. I had done as much as I needed to prove myself.

Prior to becoming disabled I was quite able to do anything I put my mind to—sew, paint, upholster, fix electrical ap-

pliances—and I could do these things in at least passable
form. If I had been prone to make comparisons between
previous accomplishments and two nonskid strips in the bathtub, I probably would have cried. But this seemed like such a
new accomplishment—another challenge met. It was something I knew I could do if only I tried and altered the procedure enough to fit my new physical status.

Not every interaction or event is as positive as the foregoing for the disabled person attempting to reestablish
himself outside of the hospital setting. Mixed emotions are
experienced when one is attempting to relearn certain things.
At some point in the early months after I became disabled I
recall that I was angry most of the time. If I tried to do
something for myself and a nondisabled person interfered, I
became angry because it seemed they did not have enough
confidence in me to think I could do things for myself. Then
at some point—a very fine line of differentiation—I grew tired
of the struggle and became angry because the others were too
insensitive to recognize that I needed help. I talked about this
dilemma with a friend and she told me that knowing how I
felt made things a lot easier for her because now she knew
there was no way she could win. She said there was no way
she could out-guess me and I would just have to take responsibility for telling her what I did and did not want her to
do. That was an excellent lesson in reality. I suddenly became
aware that I had become so self-centered and so preoccupied
with self that I expected others to magically anticipate my
every need and mood, and then behave accordingly.

The struggle the disabled person goes through is one of dependence vs. independence; not totally unlike the dependent-
independent struggle of adolescence. However, there are also
distinct differences, since the recently disabled adult has
known other levels of interaction and self-definition. Now he
not only has to resolve feelings about the loss of what once
was but he also has to learn new skills commensurate with his
abilities. He needs also to accept a greater measure of
dependence—at least in the beginning.

Another change in the disabled person's relationships comes about because significant others are not always ready, willing, or able (nor should they be expected) to adapt to the disabled person's level of capabilities. Sometimes, and understandably so, the nondisabled do not find it easy to adjust to the disabled person's slowed down pace or to the amount of extra planning that is required for the disabled person to engage in some activities. There is a period of increased sensitivity that most people with acquired disabilities go through, but the disabled must relearn to give as well as take and to realize that others also have rights and privileges. Nurses are in an excellent position to observe patient-family interactions and to intervene in instances where the family needs to be supported against acquiescing to the patient's every demand because they (the family) have not learned to cope with their grief and its associated guilt feelings. On the other hand, my friends and family have often included me on outings that I would not have gone on had it not been for their insistence and support. These issues must be mutually dealt with and reevaluated constantly if the disabled person and his family, or other companions, are to work out arrangements that are suitable to all concerned.

An able-bodied companion of a disabled person also bears the brunt of negative social attitudes toward the disabled (Davis, 1961). This may occur in various ways. For example, if I go shopping with a nondisabled friend, salespeople frequently do not speak to me directly even though I am the one about to make a purchase. I have emerged from fitting rooms carrying garments on my arm and holding my plastic money in my hand, saying to the clerk, "I want to buy these," only to have the clerk turn to my friend and say, "Did the dresses fit her? Does she want to buy them?" The first time this sort of thing happened I could not believe it! I had no preparation for this kind of response.

Early in my disability my friends became very uncomfortable in some of these situations. Not knowing what they should do, some of them tried to speak for me. This did nothing to lessen their discomfort, and I did not like to have them speak for me and reinforce the notion that I could not talk for myself. Now when such events occur, people who know me well tell the salesperson to ask me what I want. Either that, or I tell the salesperson that I am capable of speaking for myself.

Another interesting facet of this problem is that now, having been disabled for almost ten years, these incidents do not happen as frequently as they did when I was first disabled. There may be several reasons for this change: First, the new legislation regarding the disabled, especially in the area of barrier-free design, has given the disabled person greater access to stores, restaurants, and public places. Therefore, the public is more accustomed to dealing with disabled people. Second, I think I have changed in the way I present myself to others. I am not sure what has changed, but I can share with you how the change evolved.

After my initial encounters with salespeople, and others, which left me feeling like a hurt, depressed nonentity, I made up my mind that for a time I would go shopping alone. Since there was no one else to rely on I was forced to interact with salespeople, and they had to deal directly with me. I think I learned to reassert myself and to nonverbally communicate that I am a competent person. Placing nondisabled persons in the position of having to interact with the disabled person seems to be effective in breaking down the stereotypes that physical disability means that one is poor, not too bright, and possibly hard of hearing. At least I have noticed recently that people have stopped shouting at me and enunciating *very carefully* as if I somehow am not capable of hearing or understanding. I still am working on the problem of having little old ladies come up to me and ask, "Do you have arthritis, Dear?" I think they are hoping that they have found a kindred soul whose joints ache as badly as theirs do. Since most encounters now are more relaxed and natural, I am not reminded of being different as often. Therefore, grieving is minimal and increases only when there are other stresses such as a transitory illness. In rehabilitation, whether carried out by health professionals, family, or others, a necessary task is to help the disabled person learn to adapt to these kinds of encounters.

Another recurring problem for the disabled is the tendency to associate many aspects of personal encounters with their disability. Some disabled people think that others do not like them because of their disability. That may not be true. Maybe others do not like them because they have poor interpersonal skills. That may be related tangentially to their being disabled, but it is a correctable situation, given appropriate professional intervention. A recent example of this kind of association of events to one's disability took place when my husband and I went to a restaurant. This particular restaurant has a counter where people can stand or sit and have a libation while waiting for a table. I was standing and sipping a martini when I noticed a boy about three years old staring intently at my hand. I immediately assumed that he was looking at my crippled fingers and wondering what was wrong with them. I said "Hi" in order to break the ice, because, once given the opportunity, children usually can be relied upon to say what they are thinking. In this way I would be in a better position to respond. To my delight, both with the child and with my own craziness, the boy said, "Can I have your olives?"

NURSING

Reeducation for family and social roles is vital and should be included in care plans for persons with long-term illnesses or disabilities. Nurses should study carefully the methods by which these issues can be broached with the patient and his significant others. Hanson (Chapter 3) discusses sexual counseling for these patients. Cole (Green, 1975) supports the concept that sexual counseling, like other issues in the health care of the disabled, should be addressed matter-of-factly as an activity of daily living. When introducing the various and sundry topics related to activities of daily living, the health professional must be attuned to the patient's responses. In this way the health professional can become more aware of timing in introducing topics and, in addition, can also develop an increasing awareness of the depth of discussion that is appropriate for an individual at any given moment.

In one setting, I observed that some of the professional staff introduced material about the many variations possible in sexual practices without bothering to explore the patient's values, attitudes, and preferences. Frequently patients became so defensive that they resisted discussing any topic that was personal in nature. Some patients became so negatively conditioned by this premature, insensitive assault on what they considered their private domain of feelings, that other matters could not be discussed with them even when it was necessary and appropriate to do so.

There can be rather dire consequences when the foregoing type of situation occurs. Patients and their families are then poorly prepared for the patient's reentry into family and social roles. The patient leaves the hospital in a cloud of ignorance. He does not know what is or is not possible for him, and he does not know how to begin adapting to the optimum degree to any situation whether it be at a tea party or in bed.

In addition, the disabled person often needs help in learning to cope with attitudes of family and friends. The attitudes of others do not always mean rejection or overprotection, although these two reactions are quite common. Oftentimes the attitudes of significant others can best be summed up as a question, "Why did this happen to you?" These significant others are just as bewildered as is the patient about "Why?" Realistic or not, they too often wonder if their failure to pay more attention to some detail in the patient's life contributed in some way to causing the illness or disability.

Many people with long-term illnesses or disabilities have mentioned that they are often on the receiving end of questions or comments that make them feel as if they have failed their significant others by becoming ill or disabled. As my mother once said to me, "I was so proud of you when you were young. You were so alive and healthy. I wish I could change things back to the way they were." I remember asking her if she could not accept me as a cripple. In turn, she asked me if I accepted being one, to which I had to reply, "Never." She then said that she could not accept it either and added, "I still love you," as if in spite of what I had become. It took my mother four years to say what she had been thinking all that time. Appropriate anticipatory guidance on the part of nurses or other health professionals could do a great deal to prepare the disabled person for such comments and actually facilitate bringing these concerns into the open. Appropriate anticipatory guidance could also be used to teach the disabled person ways of facilitating communication about themselves so that they, in turn, could teach others how to live with them. I would have welcomed such assistance. Grief resolution is only prolonged when open discussion about these and other important feelings is avoided.

CONCLUSIONS

The important questions the helping person or agent needs to ask relate to how the disabled person can be assisted to make the necessary role modifications in order to regain optimum functioning. In this context it is important that the helping person have knowledge of social, family, and patient attitudes toward disability if the assessment and planning are to be as complete and as effective as possible.

The nurse and other health professionals should also realize that the newly disabled person grieves and goes through the many phases of grieving as described in Chapter 1. Helping the disabled person toward resolution of the grief process is an important dimension of nursing care. In order to accomplish this task, the nurse must first understand the mood swings and phase-related behaviors in the grieving process as these relate to the disabled person. Second, the nurse must be able to alter procedures and interventions to give the patient an ever increasing sense of control or mastery over life events. Such help should include preparation of the patient for the shock of reentry into a society attuned to able-bodied people. It should also include teaching the disabled person the importance of assuming personal responsibility for teaching others how to live with him; for making clear statements about needs and the kind of help that is desired from others.

REFERENCES

Byrne, D. 1961. Interpersonal attraction and attitude similarity. *Journal of Abnormal and Social Psychology* 62: 713–15.

Clore, G. L., and Jeffery, K. M. 1972. Emotional role playing, attitude change, and attraction toward a disabled person. *Journal of Personality and Social Psychology* 23:105–11.

Cogswell, B. W. 1968. Self-socialization: readjustment of paraplegics in the community. *Journal of Rehabilitation* 35:11–13.

Cole, T. M. 1975. Sexuality and the spinal cord injured. In *Human sexuality: a health practitioner's text.* ed. R. Green. Baltimore: Williams and Wilkins Company.

Comer, R. J., and Piliavin, J. A. 1972. The effects of physical deviance upon face-to-face interaction. *Journal of Personality and Social Psychology* 23:33–39.

D'Affliti, J. G., and Weitz, G. W. 1977. Rehabilitating the stroke patient through patient-family groups. *Coping with physical illness,* ed. R. H. Moos. New York: Plenum Medical Book Company.

Davis, F. 1961. Deviance disavowal: the management of strained interaction with the visibly handicapped. *Social Problems* 9:120–32.

Goffman, E. R. 1963. *Stigma: notes on the management of a spoiled identity.* Englewood Cliffs, N.J.: Prentice-Hall.

Kleck, R.; Hastorf, A. H.; and Ono, H. 1966. Emotional arousal in interactions with stigmatized persons. *Human Relations* 19:425–36.

Lewis, C. S. 1961. *A grief observed.* New York: Bantam Books.

Richardson, S. A.; Hastorf, A. H.; Goodman, N.; and Dornbusch, S. M. 1961. Cultural uniformity in reaction to physical disabilities. *American Sociological Review* 26: 241–47.

Safilios-Rothschild, C. 1970. *The sociology and social psychology of disability and rehabilitation.* New York: Random House.

Seligman, M. E. P. 1975. *Helplessness: on depression, development and death.* San Francisco: W. H. Freeman and Company.

CHAPTER THREE

Effects of Grief, Associated with Chronic Illness and Disability, on Sexuality

E. Ingvarda Hanson

INTRODUCTION

Sexuality permeates humanity. As a people of the world and of a nation, we struggle through our existence with a desperate need to bear and to care for the next generation. We are intent on leaving the world and our nation intact for children so they, too, can perpetuate man's existence. While humanity vibrates with sexual drives, sexual pleasures, and sexual frustrations, it is subjected simultaneously to great losses, natural and self-imposed, as are individuals. And humanity grieves as do individuals. Sexual experiences and grieving experiences are so entwined in the human experience that the specific effect of grief on sexuality becomes obscured. Yet within individuals this effect becomes evident particularly when grief is precipitated by the occurrence of long-term illness and disability (Schoenberg et al., 1970). The purpose of this chapter, then, is to discuss some effects of the grief response in long-term illness and disability on the sexuality of individuals, to present guidelines for nursing assessment of sexual health as it is influenced by grief, and to suggest related nursing interventions. Although the focus of this chapter is the individual and his family, community and world health concerns are not to be negated.

Sexuality encompasses the biological, physiological, psychological, and sociological components of a person that are related to that person's gender. That long-term illness and disabilities directly impinge on the "sexual system" is axiomatic; what effect the ongoing grieving process associated with long-term illness and disability has on sexuality is more obscure. The concept of self as a sexual person is vulnerable to grief, as are sexual roles, responses to sexual stimuli, and sexual relationships.

EFFECTS OF GRIEF ON SEXUAL IDENTITY AND ON ATTACHMENT

The early months of life are crucial to sexual identity development (Money and Erhardt, 1972) and the concurrent development of attachment (Bowlby, 1969). The interdependency of these two phenomena is clear. The adult who molds the sexual identity of a child by repeatedly telling the child through words and actions "you are a boy" or "you are a girl," may likely be the person with whom primary attachment develops. When associations between these highly significant early child experiences are revived in later life the person may experience a loss of secure sexual identity plus a threat to his feelings of attachment for significant others. For some persons the inevitable response to this compounded loss is to grieve.

Sexual identity, that is, knowing and feeling that one is male or female, is an ongoing presence within a person (Money and Erhardt). The small child substitutes the awareness of existing, that is, "I am," with the awareness of sexual identity, "I am a girl" or "I am a boy." Such awareness in the adult so penetrates the whole fabric of life that the person loses awareness of its presence. That is, a person usually is not concerned about sexual identity until such identity is threatened or is replaced with a new, more commanding identity—the identity of a diagnosis. When the onset of illness is abrupt and the pronouncement is made, "You have had a heart attack," "Your spinal cord is seriously injured," or "You have diabetes," the message may be translated to "I am a heart patient," or "I am a cripple," or "I am a diabetic." Each waking moment becomes a struggle between the threatened "I am Sue, a woman" or "I am John, a male," and the new identity, "I am a disease!" Although such a phenomenon may also occur in short-term illness, persons with a short, self-limiting illness are more likely to maintain personal identity; for example, the statement, "I am sick with the flu," implies a separation of self, "I am," from the illness. Therefore, many persons with a chronic illness or disability, and some with short-term illness, cannot readily integrate sexual identity and illness identity. Indeed, when sexual identity is threatened or replaced with illness identity, some individuals experience a sense of loss that may precipitate a grieving response.

Acute awareness of the loss of secure sexual identity is repeatedly experienced for some persons with chronic illness. Newly diagnosed persons may well awaken in the morning feeling wonderful and secure about themselves, when suddenly the new identity "I am an illness," crosses their mind. A dull, painful hurt envelops them as they instantaneously grieve the loss of the personal security they formerly had in knowing "I am Sue." Such grieving may indeed be momentary. It usually will be overshadowed by the overt problems of facing the day. For some even getting out of bed looms as a large problem. For others there may be constraints on diet, energy, or productivity. These latter also are losses and may precipitate grief. It is recognized, however, that other newly diagnosed persons respond to the multiple losses associated with chronic illness and to threats on their sexual identity by denying the illness and/or its effect on the sexual self. Awareness of the loss is then delayed as is the grieving process.

When sexual identity is threatened by an illness identity, several aspects of life are altered. The person may feel unable to relate to other people of the same or opposite sex because such relationships are contingent upon the individual's self-perceptions of maleness or femaleness. Both identification behavior, that is, behavior toward persons of the same sex and complementation behavior (Money and Erhardt), that is, how one relates to persons of the opposite sex, may be adversely affected when an individual sees himself as "I am an illness." Illness in Western culture is viewed by some as a state of being neuter or asexual. The neuter person can no longer rely on the lifelong patterns of identification or complementation behavior when relating to others. New patterns of behavior (that is, neuter or asexual behavior) must be developed in order to meet the expectations of society. Yet, such unnatural feelings about self create frustration. Establishing intimate relationships becomes difficult. Here begins a cycle of grieving: a perceived loss of sexual identity and the inherent loss of secure patterns of relating to others precipitates grief. The grieving process may further inhibit the person from relating to others. If a breakdown in relationships threatens significant attachments, an additional loss occurs. The cycle of grieving is perpetuated.

EFFECTS OF GRIEF ON SEX ROLE BEHAVIORS

Societies tend to view certain mannerisms, modes of dress, aspects of parenting, housework, and gainful employment, as being appropriate for a specific sex. In other words, some people not only code certain behavior as male behavior or female behavior but they also rely on these activities as the evidence of their sexual identity. Such persons, when subjected to a chronic illness that forces them to give up a sex-coded activity, are understandably threatened by the change. Additional trauma occurs when the lost activity is replaced by tasks usually associated with the opposite sex. For example, a man who has been gainfully employed outside the home may need to do the housework so that his wife can work to support them during his illness. Two losses are therefore sustained: first, the loss of the activity itself, including its rewards, and secondly, the loss of an activity that may have been significant to the individual as evidence of his or her sexuality. Compensations, such as financial aid, may be found for the first loss, but compensation is usually not possible for the second—that is, for feelings of sexual loss. When a person who lives within a family unit must alter a behavior he has coded as appropriate only to his sex, another family member usually must compensate for that change. In the traditional family situation in which a husband gives up employment because of illness, the wife may be forced to work outside the home for economic reasons. She then must also alter her housekeeping routines. Feelings of loss may be experienced by both persons. If employment and housekeeping behaviors have been significantly coded as appropriate for a specific sex by this couple, the ill husband will grieve not only for his job but also for his sexual role, as will the wife. Furthermore, in day-to-day activities, where she must become the breadwinner and he the househusband, both are constantly reminded of their loss. They are never allowed to forget or leave behind the past. The inability to carry out sexually significant behaviors while simultaneously being confronted with a cross–sex role activity is threatening and may precipitate grieving in some persons. Prolonged intense grief can demonstrate itself in various ways: through ineffective functioning in the new activity, through general feelings of sexual inadequacy, and through a reduced capacity to be responsive to the emotional and sexual needs of others (see Case Illustration II, p. 31).

When sexual identity is threatened by long-term illnesses and disabilities, sex-coded roled behavior may be used to compensate for the initial loss. With great determination, a person may try to convince the world and himself of who he is through the use of sex-coded role behaviors. Activities such as work, parenting, and recreation may take on added significance and/or become props to his threatened sexual identity. Such sex-coded role behaviors have a therapeutic effect for some persons who are grieving. Other persons, however, are faced with a compounded dilemma: a long-term illness or disability, which negatively affects sexual identity *and* which forces alterations in sex-coded role behavior, creates a dramatic loss. Grief in response to physical illness and disability is magnified as the individual must simultaneously face threatened sexual identity and altered sex-coded role behaviors. In addition, the direct adverse effect of some illnesses or disabilities on physical sexual expression must not be underestimated.

EFFECTS OF GRIEF ON PHYSICAL SEXUAL EXPRESSION

The direct effect of specific chronic illnesses and disabilities on physical expression is described in the literature (Money, 1967; Naughton, 1975; Tyler, 1976). However, in those situations where there is no direct effect between a chronic illness or disability and the sexual response cycle, an indirect effect is highly probable. Chronic illness or disability may affect love play leading to the sexual response cycle; it may affect endurance necessary for this cycle to occur; or it may affect the desire for physical sexual expression.

The effect of grief itself on the physical sexual response cycle is not clearly understood. Certainly the depressive aspect of grief has the potential to lower libido and may lead some persons to feel unworthy of pleasure, particularly sexual pleasure. Consequently, these persons might not respond to sexual stimuli within their own body nor respond when they are stimulated by a partner. When the depressive aspects of grief deter sexual drive and/or expression, some individuals will interpret their own reduced sexual interest as being a direct result of the illness or disability. If such a belief is not discussed with the health professional, the patient may readily assume that as the illness is permanent, so is loss of sexual desire. This interpretation might well deepen the grief state, which in turn will further diminish the sexual response. Gradually the sexual partner will also assume that permanent sexual dysfunction or disinterest exists. The partner's withdrawal of sexual overtures will only confirm to the patient that now he is an asexual person.

Summary. Although chronic illness and disability may directly inhibit or threaten sexual identity, sex-coded role behaviors, and physical sexual response, the effects of related grief may be equally devastating. The grieving process reduces available energy required for positive feelings about self as a sexual person, for sexual expression through sex-coded role behaviors, and for the sexual desire essential to physical expression. The resulting asexual behavior will only discourage or disenchant a potential sexual partner. Likewise, the potential partner's withdrawal may reinforce asexual feelings in the patient and perpetuate the grieving process.

NURSING ASSESSMENT OF SEXUAL HEALTH IN PERSONS EXPERIENCING GRIEF

Nursing assessment of sexual health needs in persons experiencing grief is a complex process. In fact, five major sexual health considerations must be made by the nurse as she interacts with the grieving patient for the purpose of assessment. No aspect of this assessment can be completed by a simple question and answer. Rather, the sexual health needs are identified by discussing with the patient selected aspects of his or her life. Preferably these discussions extend over a period of time. It is important to remember that sexual health assessment of the grieving patient is *not* something the nurse can do *to* the patient; instead, identification of sexual health needs evolves as the patient and nurse talk together during the process of assessment. The five areas of sexual health assessment to be considered are as follows:

1. Changes in life functions that occur as a result of a loss and the potential effect of such changes on sexuality. Chronic illnesses and disabilities inevitably alter to a greater or lesser degree major aspects of life functioning such as employment, avocations, social life, and living arrangements for the individuals affected. Most frequent changes will occur for the individual in work, recreation, housing, economic resources, and in social life. It is significant that changes in any or all of these areas have a direct effect on sexuality. Together the nurse and the patient must determine what aspects of life have changed because of the illness or what potential changes are anticipated. With a person whose work life is altered because of illness, the nurse must ascertain whether or not he associates work disability with sexual disability. For some the ability to work signifies potency, while for others the converse is true. Some feel that persons who work have the right to sexual pleasure, while those who do not work should not have that privilege. Likewise, curtailment of recreational activities, such as dancing, tennis, and so on, that provided outlets for social/sexual expression may precipitate sexual frustration. Such sexual frustration may be felt on either an emotional or physical level.

Changes in housing are needed as a result of some illnesses and disabilities. For example, the patient may need to move from a friendly, familiar environment to one that is less taxing on physical energy but nonsupportive in feeling.

Sleeping arrangements may be altered to fit the special needs of the ill person. In addition, the persons living in a household may have to move in order to accommodate the ill person. Young children may move out or a care provider, be it a family member or employee, may move into the home. Certainly those ill persons who move into extended care facilities face the most dramatic changes. When provisions for privacy and sleeping arrangements are changed an environment conducive to physical sexual expression, be it self-pleasuring or with a partner, is altered. Therefore, it becomes apparent that almost any alteration in housing has the potential to adversely affect sexuality and that nursing assessment is indicated. The nurse should consider not only what housing changes have occurred or will occur, but also the patient's perception of this change as it relates to his/her sexuality.

The loss of economic resources often associated with chronic illness and disability threatens independence. When economic dependency is forced on some individuals, a threat to sexuality is experienced. The ability to provide for self, for spouse, and for children is closely associated with masculinity even in today's liberated society. However, many women experience similar feelings of loss when their earning power is lowered. Lowered financial resources also reduce the patient's ability to purchase items that support masculinity or femininity such as fashionable clothes, hairdresser services, and exercise spas. These are examples of essential props to the sexual image of some people; indeed, the loss of such items may be devastating. It is apparent that the nurse and patient must identify the significance of an economic reversal on the individual's sexuality as well as the effect of such reversal on the patient's total well-being.

Whether a patient must face one or many changes in life functioning as a result of chronic illness or disability, feelings of great loss may follow. Even significant attachments to people can be threatened by changes in life functioning. The result for many persons is grief—a chronic grieving process for some. In such situations, the nurse must assess the extent to which the grief itself interferes with a person's ability to cope with the changes in his or her life. When grief is demonstrated by rigidity and restricted patterns of behavior, adaptation to the changes in life functioning becomes difficult. And when adaptation is adversely affected by grief, the sexual problems inherent in a change of work, recreation, housing, and economy increase.

In summary, the nurse taking part in a sexual assessment must identify which life functions have changed, or will change, as a result of illness or disability. In what way does the change directly affect the sexuality of the individual? If a grief response occurs, what is its effect on adaptation? Are the sexual concerns and problems associated with changes in life functioning exaggerated by the grief process?

2. Changes in sexual identity and sexual role. Sexual identity and sexual role are readily affected by grief. Before making an assessment of the effect of grief, however, the nurses must assess the *direct effect* of the chronic illness or disability on identity and role. Such an assessment includes several aspects. Does the patient talk about himself or herself as a masculine or feminine person *or* is the patient preoccupied with illness identity? Does the patient show concern for sexual expression, be it in modes of dress, general appearance, attractiveness to others, *or* is he engrossed in the care of his ill body as a neuter object? Is the patient concerned with personally carrying out behaviors that had previously been important to his sexual role concept such as parenting, work, and housekeeping, *or* is he concerned simply with whether or not a task is accomplished? After answering these questions about the assessment process, the nurse is ready to assess the effect of related grief on the person's sexual identity and sexual roles. The grieving process, especially when expressed in a depressive manner, may well be

demonstrated by a generalized lack of interest in one's self as a sexual person. Self-care and pride in one's appearance frequently deteriorate. Emotional investment in sex role activities is minimal. The person shows little concern for his investment in attachment relationships, and there may be a reduced concern about other persons, be it a spouse or a child. The nurse might identify that a spouse or children are neglected beyond that which the illness or disability would be expected to cause. Such behaviors suggest that grief is negatively affecting the patient's ability to carry out the behaviors that are usually associated with sexual role.

3. **Changes in sexual life style.** Assessment of sexual life style is also a consideration for the nurse. Sexual life style refers to characteristics of a person's sexual life, such as choice of love object, be it heterosexual or homosexual, and marital status. Identification of persons who are significant to the patient and who may be affected by his illness is also indicated. Although grief would not likely affect a person's choice of love object, grief could indeed affect patterns of fidelity, infidelity, or sexual liaisons. The grieving person may lose interest in significant others, including the spouse, and withdraw from previously intimate relationships. Other grieving persons may abruptly abandon partners and seek new relationships with the feeling, "The loss makes life dismal so I may as well abandon the past and 'live it up' when I can." Or, the grieving person may feel unworthy or unacceptable to those he loves. On the other hand, grieving persons sometimes seek greater closeness with their sexual partners, invest more of themselves in a union, and intensely work to enhance a relationship. Significant people may be perceived as the one constant and hopeful aspect of life.

The details of a person's sexual life style are not usually important to the nurse. Rather, the themes of a grieving person's sexual life style take on significance: (1) Has the person made major changes in his life style while grieving? (2)

If so, what effect will the changes have on his present and future life? (3) How might the significant persons be supportive to the patient? Likewise the nurse must be aware that when persons who are living with grief due to chronic illness or disability are, in addition, subjected to a change in sexual life styles created by the death of a spouse or a divorce, the effects of such loss are magnified. Certainly the person who grieves a chronic illness or disability may well have less energy available to handle the additional loss of a sexually significant person. Such an event signals the need for careful assessment of the person's capacity to cope with additional stress. The patient is vulnerable. Sexual identity and sexual roles are inevitably threatened.

4. **Changes in sexual maturity.** Sexual maturity refers to a stage or phase of sexual development that is frequently associated with chronological age. Sexual maturity is subject to stresses of physiological, emotional, or sociological origin. Loss and the resultant grief appears to significantly affect the sexual maturity of some persons. Therefore, the nurse must consider the sexual maturity of the grieving person as part of nursing assessment. Is the individual able to function at the level of sexual development usually associated with his chronological age? Inherent in this consideration is a complex issue: Has this person ever grown to his optimal sexual maturity? Has a prolonged grief reaction to a chronic illness or disability prevented such maturation? Or has a prolonged grief reaction caused the person to regress to earlier patterns of sexual behavior? The extent to which the grieving process or the illness itself precipitates the regression is difficult to determine, yet such is not the significant issue. Rather it is important to assess the patient's current level of sexual functioning—whatever the reason for such. For example, adults when confronted with the stress of a grief response may demonstrate behavior similar to that of a young adult or adolescent. Such behavior is typified by uncertainty in sexual

identity, intense concern for physical and emotional feelings associated with sexual expression, and hesitation to accept responsibility for the consequences of sexual behavior. In more intense grief responses, adults may regress to childlike sexuality; that is, they may have no erotic sensations, preferring the cuddling and holding associated with mothering care of the small child. They might lose previously strong preferences in their choice of loved object. Concerns about physical sexual expression may be denied. On the other hand, the nurse must remember that not all grieving persons revert to earlier patterns of sexual functioning; for some, sexual maturity remains a stable constant in a threatened world. Assessment of the actual level, whether it is stable or regressed, of a person's sexual maturity as evidenced by behavior rather than just his chronological age will guide the nurse as she plans for sexual health care.

5. Changes in the modes of sexual expression. "Modes of sexual expression" refers to all the behaviors that are commonly associated with sexual expression in general and specifically with the sexual response cycle. Fantasy, caressing, and intercourse are but a few examples. In fact, every person has a vast variety of modes of sexual expression available. Fantasy, for example, is not contingent upon a sound body. Seeing, hearing, talking with a loved person all serve as modes of sexual expression as do touching, holding, and all the varieties of intercourse, including the use of any body part. Sexual expression might also be experienced through creative efforts, work, and recreational pursuits. There are almost limitless varieties of modes available! Unfortunately some of the chronic illnesses and disabilities do curtail modes of sexual expression. For example, paralyzed extremities deter masturbation or the holding and caressing of another person. A few illnesses and disabilities directly interfere with the physiological sexual response cycle. Other illnesses limit social encounters, thereby restricting intimate relationships from forming. Grief, however, appears to have no direct effect upon the physiological aspects of the sexual response cycle; nevertheless, grief may diminish enjoyment or alter the physiological sexual response cycle because of its impact upon the emotions. Both the grieving person and the significant other are vulnerable to these adverse effects.

Assessment of physical sexual functioning during illness and disability centers on whether or not, under any circumstances, erections or pelvic engorgement and vaginal lubrication occur. Knowledge of the anatomical injury or lesion may help in predicting whether or not physical sexual functions will return. Of greater importance, however, is the significance that the patient attaches to the affected or lost mode of sexual expression. The nurse must help the patient refocus by having him/her identify the modes of sex expression that remain intact, that are acceptable (that is, morally approved by the patient), and that are significant to him or her.

To what extent the grieving process itself adversely affects enjoyment of the modes of sexual expression is more difficult to assess. The nurse should explore with the patient the changes that have occurred in his enjoyment of sexual expression since the onset of the illness or disability, then speculate with the patient upon the cause for these changes. Some changes could easily be explained by physical pathology, others by the restrictions of the environment. However, if additional changes remain unexplained, one might assume that the grieving process itself is draining energy from creative sexual expression. The grieving patient might identify vague concerns such as, "I just don't care about sex any more." Some patients may disclose that they are hesitant to pursue physical sexual expression for fear of failure or disappointment and thereby face another loss. An opposite behavior may be described by others. They intently pursue new modes of sexual expression in a desperate attempt to hide, deny, or obliterate intense feelings of loss that accompany grief. Nursing assessment of the effect that grief has on modes of sexual expression includes not only a consideration of the direct effect of the illness or disability, but also identification of the additional changes that may be attributed to the grieving process.

Summary. Sexual assessment of the person who is experiencing grief is not a simple question and answer procedure. The nurse and patient must discuss the changes in the patient's life that he perceives as having an effect on his sexuality. Of special concern are changes in sexual identity, sex-coded behaviors, sexual life style, sexual maturity, and the modes of sexual expression. Although it is difficult through the process of assessment to implicate grief as *the* cause for adverse changes, the nurse will be able to identify the major sexual health concerns if she thoroughly considers the five aspects of assessment.

NURSING INTERVENTION RELATED TO SEXUAL HEALTH

In sexual health care, nursing assessment, planning, and intervention are usually entwined. This is particularly true when nursing a grieving person. Assessment, planning for care, and the actual provision of sexual health care cannot be relegated to a limited time period if a meaningful intervention is to occur. The first consideration for nursing intervention, that of communicating about sexuality, includes the assessment process. It is the nurse who must tell the patient that sexual concerns are real, legitimate, and to be discussed openly whenever the patient is ready to do so. Such information, when given with tact and in a manner that asks nothing of the patient, may serve to reduce embarrassment or guilt about having sexual concerns. As the nurse discusses changes that have occurred in the patient's life as a result of the illness, disability, and grieving process, she will introduce whatever questions are pertinent: Which of these changes may affect your feelings of masculinity/femininity? Which will affect your feelings as a sexual person? As a sexual partner? As a parent? In the discussion of these and related assessment questions, the nurse will help the patient recognize for himself areas of sexual concern with which he will need assistance, as well as areas that he can handle with his own resources. The grieving person then is encouraged to share feelings about specific sexual losses in his life and to put them into the perspective of himself as a whole person and as a family member. Eventually the nurse will discuss the resources available to help the patient minimize each of the sexual losses experienced.

Sexual education is also a part of nursing intervention for the grieving person. Knowledge of and direction in the use of one's body for sexual expression may provide a previously unexplored source of pleasure to a person experiencing a deficit of such experiences. Sex education helps the individual expand his perception of sex-coded role behaviors. Such insight permits the patient to find alternative role behaviors and it helps him understand his family's reactions to sex-coded behavior change. Other persons will need assistance as they transfer information about their illness or disability and grief to the area of sexuality. For example, while a patient may understand that the lack of energy is related to grief, he might not understand that lowered energy may be the cause of his reduced sexual desire.

Nursing intervention related to sexuality also includes family education. The nurse, with patient consent, should share with the spouse or sexual partner information on the sexual implications of chronic illness and disability and of inherent grief. Open discussion with the patient and significant others on their joint sexual concerns will help to explode myths, facilitate communication, and, therefore, promote sexual health.

Nursing care, which promotes enhanced feelings about self as a sexual person and which promotes social and intimate relationships with significant others, is imperative. The nurse should minimize the patient's physical discomfort that could detract from his sexual feelings. Privacy, cleanliness, and good grooming enhance sexuality. Individualized nursing care plans are essential. In-depth discussions between nurse and patient about the possible effects of grief on sexuality and the significance of that effect on the patient are also part of the therapeutic interventions. Such discussions will facilitate the patient's movement through the grieving process.

Nurses with even minimal preparation in sexual health care can make a major contribution to the professional team by sharing their assessments and ideas about the implementation of such care. However, when nurses assess that a patient has a major physical change or psychological problem involving grief that taxes the patient's ability to cope with related sexual changes in his life, referral is indicated. Indeed, referral then becomes part of the nursing intervention. A physician and/or nurse therapist may be needed to treat those major physical and emotional sexual problems that are compounded or precipitated by grief. However, a referral to sexual dysfunction therapy as such is usually delayed until physical care and emotional help with the loss itself has been given. Fortunately, on many occasions sexual health problems will resolve when the patient's general physical and emotional health improves. It is important to recognize that nursing referral to other sexual health care professionals does not absolve the nurse from further responsibility for sexual health care. In cooperation with the primary therapist, the nurse can support whatever plan of care will facilitate the patient's effective use of therapy.

Ongoing evaluation of nursing assessment, planning, and intervention is particularly essential when working with the person who experiences grief associated with chronic illness or disability. Such is true because each day a new situation may precipitate or renew a loss experience. Plans and intervention methods used yesterday, therefore, might not be applicable today. Sex education needs are quickly outmoded. Referrals need alteration. Fresh insights into the effects of grief on sexuality may be forthcoming. The effects of drugs, X-ray, physical therapy, or psychotherapy on the patient's sexuality must constantly be appraised. Such constant, ongoing evaluation cannot be done independent of the health team. More importantly, it cannot be done without frequent input from the patient and his family. Ordinarily the patient will be able to evaluate what aspect of his sexuality and to what extent his sexuality is affected by the ever fluctuating grieving process. The patient will know when therapies have lifted the weight of grief from his feelings about himself as a sexual person, his sexual role pleasures and conflicts, and from his modes of sexual expression. Also, the patient's sexual partner is likely to sense improvement in the patient's ability to enjoy sexual expression as the grief is reduced. At times it will be appropriate to include the sexual partner in discussions about the sexual changes that the patient is experiencing; however, such joint evaluation is appropriate only if the patient has first agreed to include the sexual partner. Nursing assessment, planning, and implementation of sexual health care for the grieving person without evaluation is meaningless or even detrimental. Ongoing evaluation is essential to the total plan of care and will help the nurse maintain both sensitivity to the grieving patient and objectivity to his sexual health needs.

The extent to which a nurse assesses a patient's sexual health care needs associated with grieving will vary from nurse to nurse. The depth of preparation for sexual assessment differs in nursing education programs that prepare first level staff nurses from those that prepare clinical specialists. In addition, even similar programs of nursing education are frequently dissimilar in the area of sexual health care content presented. Perhaps a greater influence than the educational program per se on a nurse's ability to provide sexual health care is her own comfort with sexuality.

Although not all nurses will have either the preparation or personal comfort to assess all five areas suggested above, most nurses can contribute some observations to the health care team who, by sharing with each other, will make a thorough assessment. Likewise, nurses will provide different levels of sexual health intervention. Most, if not all, nurses should as a minimum promote a milieu respectful of the patient's sexuality. Nurse practitioners with expertise in sexual health care will make complete sexual assessments and plan for and provide therapeutic intervention. They will assist the patient to cope with sexual problems and will facilitate the patient's movement toward healthier patterns of sexual behavior.

REFERENCES

Bowlby, J. 1969. *Attachment and loss, volume 1: attachment.* New York: Basic Books, Inc., Publishers.

Bowlby, J. 1973. *Attachment and loss, volume 2: separation, anxiety and anger.* New York: Basic Books, Inc., Publishers.

Money, J. 1967. Sexual problems of the chronically ill. In *Sexual problems, diagnosis and treatment in medical practice,* ed. C. W. Wahl. New York: The Free Press.

Money, J., and Erhardt, A. 1972. *Man and woman, boy and girl.* New York: A Mentor Book, New American Library.

Naughton, K. 1975. Effect of chronic illness on sexual performance. *Medical aspects of human sexuality,* October.

Schoenberg, B.; Carr, A. C.; Peretz, D.; and Kutscher, A. K. 1970. *Loss and grief: psychological management in medical practice.* New York: Columbia University Press.

Tyler, E. A. 1976. Sex and medical illness. In *The sexual experience,* eds. B. J. Sadock, H. I. Kaplan, and A. M. Freedman. Baltimore: Williams and Wilkins Company.

ADDITIONAL BIBLIOGRAPHY

The following books are suggested readings to enhance the nurse's understanding of sexuality and sexual health care. They do not directly address the topic of the effect of grief on sexuality.

Adelson, E. T. 1975. *Sexuality and psychoanalysis.* New York: Brunner/Mazel, Publishers.

Green, R. 1975. *Human sexuality: a health practitioner's text.* Baltimore: Williams and Wilkins Company.

Green, R. 1974. *Sexual identity conflict in children and adults.* New York: Basic Books, Inc., Publishers.

Group for the Advancement of Psychiatry. 1974. *Assessment of sexual function: a guide to interviewing.* New York: Jason Aronson.

Masters, W. H., and Johnson, V. E. 1966. *Human sexual response.* Boston: Little, Brown and Company.

Kaplan, H. S. 1974. *The new sex therapy.* New York: Brunner/Mazel Publishers.

Money, J. and Tucker, P. 1975. *Sexual signatures.* Boston: Little, Brown and Company.

Sadock, B. J.; Kaplan, H. I.; and Friedman, A. M., 1976. *The sexual experience.* Baltimore: Williams and Wilkins Company.

Woods, N. F. 1975. *Human sexuality in health and illness.* St. Louis: C. V. Mosby Company.

Vincent, C. E. 1973. *Sexual and marital health: the physician as a consultant.* New York: McGraw-Hill Book Company.

Zubin, J., and Money, J. 1973. *Contemporary sexual behavior: critical issues in the 1970s.* Baltimore: Johns Hopkins University Press.

PART TWO

In Part Two, examples of three clinical and life states are addressed. Because we wanted to avoid some of the redundancy that comes with applying the concepts of grief and its resolution to specific conditions and diagnostic states, a decision was made to include an example of grief brought on by an acute physical illness, by the birth of a defective child, and by the process of aging, thinking that these three examples would touch upon major events across the age continuum.

Chapter 4, "Loss of Heart," discusses the physiological and psychological impact of acquired heart disease. Basic questions about personality typology and health prior to and following the onset of heart disease are discussed. The importance of family and work roles in grief resolution for the individual with heart disease are stressed. Concepts related to crisis intervention are included.

Chapter 5, "Grief in Parents of a Child with a Birth Handicap," is the clearest example given of grief responses in family members when there is an associated illness or disability in another of its members. In this chapter, the child is mentioned only in so far as it is the stimulus for the grief that the parents experience. Grief and grief resolution are approached from a stress-oriented model, but the reader will be able to identify behaviors that fit into the attachment theory framework as set down in Chapter 1.

Chapter 6, "Grief and the Process of Aging," examines what is inevitable for all of us who live to the point of retirement and beyond. Variations along the continuum from the well-adjusted elderly to those who react with excessive grief to losses brought on by aging are explored. Factors promoting adaptation to aging are discussed and suggestions made for nursing interventions.

CHAPTER FOUR

Loss of Heart

Mary Delaney-Naumoff

INTRODUCTION

The first realistic confrontation with mortality often occurs with the onset of acquired heart disease. Typically, these people are between the ages of forty and fifty with no previous history of major illness requiring hospitalization; although history of treatment for diabetes, hypertension, or peptic ulcer is not uncommon. Their personality characteristics are those of type A exhibiting coronary-prone behavior, that is, extremely competitive, striving for success, impatient, restless, very alert, and intelligent (Jenkins, 1971, p. 244). These people feel a great sense of urgency and pressure regarding their commitments and responsibilities. Individuals with coronary-prone behavior tend to have elevated triglyceride and cholesterol values, hyperinsulinemic response to glucose challenge, and increased diurnal secretion of norepinephrine (Jenkins et al., 1974).

Type A individuals are found in every stratum of society. This behavior is not confined only to white collar workers, nor are these characteristics confined only to men. Increasing numbers of premenopausal women are also succumbing to acquired heart disease (Moriyama et al., 1971). Postmeno-pausal women almost equal men in numbers of heart attacks per thousand population in the 55–75 year age group.

Pain in the chest is usually the first overt sign that forces a type A personality to recognize that he or she may have heart disease, but perception of symptoms does not necessarily mean the immediate seeking of medical help. Moss et al. (1969) have emphasized three distinct cognitive functions required in the decision to seek medical aid: (1) *perception* of the symptom, (2) *recognition* of the seriousness of the symptom, and (3) *realization* that medical care is indicated. The behavioral responses that may inhibit symptom recognition and continue long after diagnosis may be varied, but the dominant underlying emotion is grief. Grief is defined in the *Random House Dictionary* as: "Personal feelings experienced at the perceived loss of function, control, or ability. Keen mental suffering or distress over affliction or loss; sharp sorrow, painful regret."

The person grieves deeply because his heart, that realistic symbol of life and longevity has shown vulnerability. The heart's vulnerability has forced an individual's confrontation with death. Until now he has taken his body for granted, worked long hours, striven for success, and denied feelings of increased pressure and fatigue. His career and life goals were planned and appeared attainable; suddenly, he has lost control.

The feeling of loss is all the more acute because every patient who suffers from angina pectoris or myocardial infarction (M.I.) is very aware of friends or relatives so afflicted. The patient remembers those who died of heart disease and those who never recovered sufficiently to be able to return to an active working and social life. Those who suffered an M.I. and successfully returned to the mainstream of life are forgotten. Successful coping with the nonvisibility of heart disease removes it from the awareness of others.

Patients with heart disease anticipate the loss of their ability to work, to be supportive and functional members of their families and social groups, and, ultimately, of their lives. The change of role from independence to dependency is an additional burden patients cope with poorly.

The individual with arteriosclerotic heart disease in the acute stage of grief is probably best described by Dante in his Divine Comedy:

> Midway in the journey through life, I found myself lost in a dark wood strayed from the true path.

The patient feels he has lost power, direction, and goals—behaviors that characterize the mature adult in his interactions with others. Rather than feeling that he is in the center of activity, he feels pushed to the periphery. He becomes an outsider dependent upon the ministrations of others. These feelings of isolated dependency and depression persist throughout the acute stages of illness and into the period of convalescence and rehabilitation (Tibblin et al., 1972).

The feeling that life is over when a heart attack occurs is not just confined to the patient. This attitude may persist among health care professionals as well. A story is told that aptly illustrates the characteristic feelings experienced by patient and physician when coping with heart disease. Several years ago a patient was referred to a cardiologist for consultation. The patient had sustained a M.I. several weeks previously, and he had several questions regarding the many restrictions his own physician had placed upon him. He said to the cardiologist, "My doctor said that I must give up smoking, business, golf, sexual relations, and go to bed each night before eleven. Is that correct?" The cardiologist agreed that it was sound advice. "If I follow it," the patient said, "will I live longer?" "That," the cardiologist replied, "I can't say, but it will seem longer."

Today, with increased knowledge of cardiac physiology and pathophysiology, most of the physical limitations imposed on a patient are of a temporary nature. These limitations are gradually lifted as the rehabilitative program progresses. However, the attitude expressed in the above story has been less responsive to change. The man or woman with cardiac disease has a tendency to focus on the restrictions rather than on available options and goals to be attained.

We, as nurses, often unknowingly promote this negative focus. In our zeal to help the patient understand the seriousness of heart disease, we emphasize the need to return to the normal activities of daily living on a *gradual* basis if recovery is to proceed smoothly. We realize we are working with dynamic individuals who are not only unaccustomed to serious illness, but also may be overtly denying that illness. It is understandable then, that we emphasize activity prohibitions hoping to prevent a relapse. However, in so doing we reinforce the patient's underlying grief and growing sense of loss. If the nurse succeeds in breaking a patient's overt denial pattern, she must also be equally ready to assist him in coping with the surfacing grief and its accompanying depression.

The patient's sense of loss and helplessness may be further complicated by an increasing feeling of guilt. This is accomplished by the emphasis placed on all of the good health habits that the patient must now employ. As the nurse discusses posthospital convalescence and the desired goals of reaching optimal weight, regular exercise, and hours, as well as giving up smoking and possibly excessive drinking along with required dietary modifications, the patient will feel guilty for not having done these things prior to hospitalization. There is nothing the nurse can do to prevent this feeling of guilt which is solidly based in reality. What the nurse can do is be aware of its presence and assist the patient in using his guilt positively rather than permitting it to further compound his grief and depression.

The nurse should also be aware that some of the grieving

and depression following the onset of heart disease may be an acute manifestation of an individual's feelings about himself prior to his illness. There are many underlying concerns that a middle-aged man or woman will have that now become the focus of their attention. Very basic questions, such as:

1. The purpose of their life.
2. The realistic nature of their goals.
3. Their job future and satisfaction.
4. The future of a marriage when the children are grown.
5. Retirement.
6. Sexual virility and/or desirability.

If these questions have been nagging at the back of a patient's mind prior to his illness, they now become the central theme of his ruminations.

The possibility exists that the patient has become bored with his present career and welcomes the opportunity for a rest. "But," they ask, "will I have the energy or the time to develop an alternative?" If the marriage or sexual identity prior to the onset of illness were shaky, the nurse cannot expect these areas to be stable while the patient is ill. What the nurse must do is carefully assess which problems were caused by the illness and which problems have been exaggerated by the illness. Only with this careful assessment can the nurse expect to intelligently and effectively plan her interventions and referrals.

Family role reversal may be the most devastating of all events for some patients. Although the role change may be of a temporary nature, that is, the wife returning to work during a husband's convalescence, or another family member temporarily assuming household tasks while a wife recovers, the patient may feel permanently displaced. If the patient's sexual identity was in need of constant reinforcement based upon the family role assumed, and this role is no longer open to him, he will experience anxiety, depression, and the feeling of uselessness. The patient's perceived loss of role within the family serves to generate a perception within him that he has now become a great burden.

An illustration may be to the point. The cardiology group with which this writer was associated was asked to see a patient recently admitted to a coronary care unit. The patient had sustained a major infero–lateral wall infarct and was critically ill with early signs of cardiogenic shock. He survived this crisis and the nurse clinician began planning his convalescence program with the cardiologist, patient, and family. Upon discharge the major question in the cardiologist's mind was whether the patient was developing a ventricular aneurysm at the site of the infarct. The major concern of the patient was how soon could he return to work. For his wife and two teenage children, they questioned whether they would lose their home, friends, and the opportunity for further education. The role of the nurse was to correlate these questions and the unstated goals behind them, namely,

1. Prevention of an acute episode of pump failure (M.D.).
2. Sufficient health to return to work (Patient).
3. Social status and economic security (Family).

Could the goals of health care and those of the patient and family be accomplished? Could a compromise be reached that would be acceptable to all concerned?

This patient was the son of an Eastern European immigrant. He had left school at age 14 to help support his parents and his younger brother and sisters. As a young man he became an independent trucker, belonged to the union, and had developed a successful business. He was now 49 years of age.

About two months prior to his infarct he purchased a new truck costing about $35,000. As an independent trucker he had no sick leave benefits, was not eligible for his pension, and was responsible for the payments on his truck and for a new home in an affluent suburb. No money was coming in and he felt everyone was dependent upon him. He had a home, wife, children, and business, but he was unable to fulfill his obligations.

The nurse, aware of his background and his present feelings regarding his illness and pressing obligations, devised the following plan of care:

1. Make a home visit within the first week following discharge from the hospital to:
   a. assess the patient's physical and emotional status.
   b. discuss the patient's diet and medication regimen with him and his wife and make modifications where necessary.
   c. listen to the problems and/or questions that had arisen since the patient returned home and offer suggestions, alternatives, or make the necessary referrals.
   d. increase the patient's activities if he is physically and emotionally ready.
2. Discuss with the cardiologist the posthospital assessment of the patient and family, and further modify the plan of care as necessary.

The first home visit by the nurse revealed that the patient was progressing physically and at the present time the family was not under severe financial strain. Emotionally, however, the patient was very depressed. He cried easily, had difficulty getting to sleep, and would awaken between four and five o'clock in the morning. He hated the strict dietary regimen and "taking all those pills." The patient felt helpless, hopeless, and desperate. During the visit he said, "The children have no father, my wife has no husband, and I am no longer a man. I can do nothing anymore. Even my father at 87 can still climb on a roof to repair it."

Over the next two months the patient's physical health improved gradually but his feelings of helplessness persisted. Because of the seriousness of his infarct, the cardiologist informed him that he eventually could return to work, but on a very limited basis. Although a psychiatric referral was recommended by the nurse, neither the family nor the physician wished to pursue it. This story should have a happy ending; it does not. Three months after the onset of his infarct the patient returned to work full time, contrary to the advice of his doctor and the wishes of his family. He died in the cab of his truck after he pulled off to the side of the road. As his wife told us afterwards, the only thing he was certain of was that in death his insurance would pay for the house and the truck. Alive, as a semi-invalid, he felt he was only a burden.

This graphic illustration of unresolved grief, depression, and the economics of catastrophic illness in a family is not atypical. The family may have been unique, but the problem is not. A man works and supports his family. If he cannot work "he is not a man." This man felt he had no other options. To deprive a person of work is to remove one of the most important controls in his life (Lidz, 1968).

THE PROBLEM OF ILL HEALTH

Ill health for young or old is not easy. For the middle-aged with type A personalities, it is a source of extreme frustration. Their responses to extreme frustration are fear and hostility (Glass, 1976).

For some, there may have been a previous diagnosis of hyperlipidemia, hypertension, and/or hyper- or hypoinsulinemia. These patients were prescribed a diet or medication to which they may not have adhered. In most instances noncompliance is an indication of not being able to fit the medical regime into their life style rather than a conscious rejection of its necessity. These patients, on the other hand, are usually very conscientious regarding their family's medical care.

Glass (1976) has shown in his study, *Stress and Coronary Prone Behavior,* that persons with type A personalities respond poorly over time to constant stress. Their initial response is to work hard, suppress feelings, and ignore fatigue. When the stressor continues unchanged by their actions they become apathetic. People with type A behavior have a great need to master and control their environment. When met with a situation beyond control, due to circumstances external or internal to themselves, they become helpless and frustrated. Physiologically, serum cholesteral and norepinephrine values are elevated. Raab (1966) has indicated the specificity of norepinephrine discharge in the presence of aggression and hostility. Frustration is rarely accompanied by hostility alone. Fear and/or anxiety are also a part of the emotional complex. The physiologic response to fear is increased epinephrine secretion.

Glass pointed out in his study that significant loss or uncontrollable losses within the year would most likely lead to a heart attack in a person with type A behavior. It has also been the experience of many physicians and nurses, who work closely with patients who have cardiovascular disease, that uncontrollable stressors may lead to angina pectoris. Patients often wait until they feel a myocardial infarction is imminent before presenting themselves for care. The well-established pattern of ignoring discomfort even applies to the symptom of chest pain.

Nitroglycerin, a common prescription for angina, often is not taken by the patient. When asked the reason, a typical patient response is: "If I sit and rest a while, the pain goes away, then I can continue what I was doing," or, "The nitro gives me a slight headache or makes me feel lightheaded so that I have to wait fifteen or twenty minutes before I can continue what I was doing." These responses are true, but there is another reason why nitroglycerin may not be taken as prescribed. Taking medication removes some of the control a patient has over his body and activities. If he could overcome fatigue and discomfort through rest in the past, why can't he overcome angina as well?

The combination of uncontrolled personal loss and chest pain may produce a chronic state of frustration. The resulting anxiety and hostility, because of frustration, significantly increase catecholamine discharge, causing further oxygen depletion in an already compromised myocardium.

There is clinical and experimental evidence beyond reasonable doubt that anger and anxiety lead to the local liberation of norepinephrine within the myocardium and epinephrine from the adrenal medulla (Raab, 1966). These catecholamines cause myocardial oxygen depletion by increasing the cellular metabolic rate and heart rate while decreasing effective cardiac output. In the presence of compromised coronary arteries, due to atheromatous plaques, the consequence may be the pain of angina or the onset of infarction. The following case history illustrates this point.

A 39-year-old man was referred to our cardiology group because of increasing anginal attacks during the past year. Two years earlier he had been diagnosed as an insulin dependent diabetic. The patient had been prescribed NPH U80 insulin 35 units daily and a diabetic diet. He faithfully took his insulin but marginally adhered to his diet. He did not test his urine and was experiencing an increasing number of hypoglycemic attacks that he countered by eating candy bars. Within the previous year he suffered a large investment loss, had been involved in a legal action, and one of his children was also diagnosed as diabetic. The onset of his angina roughly corresponded to his investment loss and the initiation of the lawsuit. The frequency and duration of the anginal attacks had significantly increased within the previous three months along with his hypoglycemia. The lawsuit was soon to go to court. The patient was diagnosed as having pre-infarction angina (Prinzmetals) and was admitted to the hospital. Shortly after admission he sustained a myocardial infarction. The most significant thing he could tell us during succeeding interactions were related to the anger and frustration he felt over the events of the past year. He stated he felt his body was falling apart; that it was not allowing him to do what was necessary to provide support for his family. Now, with a heart attack plus his business and legal problems, he envisioned his family left without financial security and being held responsible for his investment losses. The patient even said he had bargained with God. If he did everything that was therapeutically indicated for his recovery, would God leave him here long enough to see that his family was secure?

Kubler-Ross (1969) has indicated that bargaining is part of the grieving process, usually following frustration and anger. The patient, in the midst of grief and depression, felt the only avenue left to gain control of his life was to bargain with God. For in thinking himself in a position to bargain, the patient felt more in control of the situation—control so necessary to the type A personality.

The purpose of this case history is to illustrate the intimate relationship between an individual's emotional state and physical response. If we, as nurses, do not assist patients in coping with grief effectively, we cannot hope to accomplish the physical goals of health care. To assist patient and family in resolving the problem of ill health is to assist in helping them work through the physical and emotional problems that accompany it. This is the first step in the resolution of grief.

LOSS OF CONTROL

The problem of ill health is inextricably tied to the loss of control. This is evident in the preceding statements. What has not been discussed is the family's response, which may increase the patient's feeling of lost control.

Denial of the seriousness of their condition is a common patient response. Denial is used as a mechanism to avoid acknowledging ill health and therefore, loss of bodily function. Initial denial is a necessary and healthy response providing the patient and family with an emotional respite. During this period of denial and relative serenity, catecholamine discharge decreases, therefore minimizing further myocardial damage. Rest is also promoted in the absence of emotional turmoil. It is not uncommon for euphoria to follow the initial crisis in the sense that patient and family agree that "everything is going to be all right." Tension eases and relaxation begins. The decrease in catecholamine discharge is evidenced by a decrease in heart rate and an increase in blood pressure to near normal levels. In some patients even cardiac arrythmias decrease or cease altogether. The patient sleeps restfully for longer periods of time.

The response may be considered unhealthy if the family participates in the patient's denial system and convince themselves that it was "just a little indigestion" or "a muscle spasm." The patient may then attempt to engage in activities that he is physically incapable of handling.

For example, a man was admitted to a coronary care unit in a large medical center. He had sustained a serious inferior wall infarct and suffered pain for a seventy-two hour period. On the fourth hospital day he was pain free and had slept well the night before. He bribed the orderly, whom he knew, to buy him a package of cigarettes. When the patient thought no one was looking and morning rounds were over, he walked into the bathroom and began smoking a cigarette. The lead cords on the cardiac monitors were ten to twelve feet long, so this action could be accomplished easily without disturbing the leads. What he didn't know, of course, was the effect that the sudden increase in activity and the nicotine were having on the rate and rhythm of his heart. The nurse quickly discovered him, put him back to bed, and confiscated the cigarettes. The patient's family was upset, but their only comment was that they could never do anything about his smoking anyway. The patient was questioned as to whether he understood that he had suffered a serious heart attack. He answered, "Look, I know you have rules for all of the patients in here, but there are always exceptions—and I am one of those exceptions!"

The above incident is extreme, though true. It clearly illustrates both the patient's need to control and the unhealthy effects of denial. The family's mild response only reinforced the patient's denial system. Many patients attempt to get out of bed as soon as the pain subsides. It doesn't matter that a commode is ordered for them or that they are told they will begin to have chair privileges the next day. It is the need to make decisions and have control of their own bodies and life styles that governs their behavior.

The family's participation in the patient's denial system is not the only harmful mechanism apparent in a patient-family relationship. The family may unwittingly increase and prolong the patient's state of anxiety by communicating their own fears. The family has every reason to be anxious, but it is the responsibility of the coronary care staff to assist the family in expressing their anxiety to the appropriate people. If the nursing staff succeed in helping the family express their anxiety to each other, a close friend, or a clergyman, the family will be less likely to communicate great anxiety to the patient. In patient-family communication, care and concern are always appropriate and therapeutic. Obvious fear is not. There is nothing communicated more rapidly in an intensive care unit than anxiety, and it is this writer's belief that nonverbal communication of anxiety is more devastating than the verbal expression of care and concern.

Clinical evidence is abundant to illustrate a patient's physiologic response to a visit from a tearful, tense, and anxious family. Heart rate and arrythmias increase and blood pressure drops. A family's fearful communication of possibly losing their loved one and their own security and control may cause the patient untold damage both physically and emotionally. The behavior of the patient's spouse, for example, may reinforce his anxiety, dependence, and invalidism or impel the patient to engage in activities that are harmful to his health and recovery (Freedman et al., 1976).

One of the most effective ways of dealing with overt and covert anxiety in patient and spouse is by confrontation. Ask them directly about their anxieties and dispel the myths and misconceptions that may form the basis of their concerns. In addition, the nursing staff should positively reinforce the benefits of rehabilitation and physical reconditioning. Positive attitudes on the part of the staff toward rehabilitation will do more to improve the patient's coping mechanisms than almost any other type of intervention.

Consistently high levels of anxiety on the part of the "well spouse" provides another area of concern for the nursing staff in coronary care. The health and well-being of the well spouse may be in jeopardy. He or she experiences great insecurity, loss of control, and helpless frustration, as does the patient. It is not uncommon for the spouse, in an acute attack of anxiety, to develop somatic symptoms similar to those of his or her mate. This writer can recall two instances in which the supposedly well spouses actually developed myocardial infarcts very similar to those of their mates. Stress, precipitating a massive neuroendocrine response (i.e., catecholamine discharge), caused myocardial ischemia and infarction.

The relationship between the patient and his family is so important that their combined attitudes may determine the rate of recovery and the degree of rehabilitation. The family's attitude may either enhance dependence and disability or lead to premature return to work and sexual activity. The patient may feel pushed to the extreme of minimizing symptoms or, conversely, of never returning to work again.

The family, as well as the patient, will experience anger, betrayal and guilt over their loss of control as the result of ill health. Anger may be directed toward the patient as much as toward themselves. The feeling of "how could he do this to us," is often expressed as "He can't die, he can't die," or "Please get better, you can't leave us now!" If the patient is still in the denial stage of his illness and acts contrary to written orders, the family may become overtly angry with the patient, "Don't you want to get well?"; or they may combine it with a little guilt, "Don't you care about us?" The patient presents the symptoms, but he must be treated as part of a disrupted family.

CRISIS RESPONSE

According to Caplan (1964), and Langsley and Kaplan (1968), the concept of crisis includes developmental transitions having the potential either for pathology or improved health and altered personal relationships. To understand the meaning of a crisis requires paying attention to the biological functioning and psychodynamics of the individual and also to explicit assessment of the social milieu; especially the family as a social system.

The phases of crisis have been described throughout the literature of psychology and sociology. It is generally agreed that there are four stages: (1) impact, (2) turmoil, (3) mobilization of resources, and (4) reconstruction. The nurse who understands crisis theory sees these stages as the expression of grief as well as the method that the patient and family use to ultimately resolve grief. Crisis theory provides another means of assessing a patient and family biologically as well as psychodynamically. The nurse who is able to assess accurately has the data necessary to create a sound management plan and to evaluate that plan.

Grief is an acute emotion, usually of sudden onset precipitated by loss of life or function. The first phase of crisis— impact—describes the psychobiological response of the patient and family to the acute onset of heart disease and their initial grief reaction.

In the first phase of crisis the emergency fight or flight pattern of behavior is mobilized. The patient is admitted to the coronary care unit with all of the symptoms of massive sympathetic discharge, which include cold sweaty palms, dilated pupils, and racing pulse, which is sometimes accompanied by arrythmia and low or dropping blood pressure. The patient is pale, often nauseated, and extremely weak. Moreover, he may appear disoriented, confused, and unable to relate what has happened to him.

The family may also be in the same state of shock. The more unexpected the patient's symptoms, usually the greater the degree of distress and shock in his family.

On the other hand, there may be the appearance of calm on the part of the patient. Depending upon his need to control, he may seem to listen and appear to understand the explanations about his condition and the physical equipment in his room. How, then, does the nurse assess the degree of physical and emotional shock present in this patient and his family? First, the physiologic parameters of shock will be present. Second, after an appropriate period of rest, ask the patient and his family what they understood of the explanations given them. In the majority of cases little of the proffered explanations will have been comprehended. In some instances patient and/or family may have forgotten completely that any discussion occurred at all. In the acute stage of shock learning cannot take place.

The period of time that patient and family remain in shock is variable. It may be hours to days in duration. The responsibility lies with the staff of the coronary care unit to assist patients and families through this difficult period as soon as possible. Prolongation of shock will only prove more destructive, physically and emotionally, for patient and family.

How often have we witnessed the continuance of pain long after a large dose of a narcotic has been administered, or the extension of infarcts in a twenty-four to forty-eight hour period following initial onset? One significant variable to be considered is the prolongation of adrenergic discharge due to shock and fear. Narcotics cannot replace the assurance of a knowledgeable, compassionate human being.

If there is anything a patient and family in crisis do not want, it is to be left alone with their fear. Regardless of what is verbalized, their contact with reality may be through the warmth of another's hand. The family need to feel the competence, comfort, and trust of the professional touch. The professional who spends five or ten minutes with the patient and family in calm activity or quiet sitting will greatly allay their anxiety. Then, a narcotic given for pain will take effect.

Coronary Care Units can be very busy places and sometimes their activity is greatly increased by the contagion of anxiety. If each nurse would spend a calm, quiet period with every new patient, the communication of that anxiety could be greatly reduced. Those few minutes may have the potential of preventing much more time spent in crisis intervention later on.

As patient and family begin to recover from the first phase of grieving and crisis they move into phase two—turmoil. A flood of emotions is experienced in which their previous coping mechanisms are no longer effective. Anxiety continues but it is now accompanied by rage, guilt, and depression. The possibility of permanent loss of the previous level of health is acutely perceived by the patient. The patient may express in one form or another the attitude of "why me?" He experiences a diffuse rage at his body's betrayal, expressing that not only did he not want a heart attack, but he didn't deserve one. As one patient stated, "I think someone doesn't like me!" The patient's anger may then turn on the doctors and nurses caring for him. Doctors and nurses are constant reminders to the patient that he is ill, dependent, and reliant on them for his well-being. The quiet "good" patient of the day before may become an angry, rude, crusty individual who cannot be made comfortable. If the nursing staff does not understand the dynamics of this stage of grief, then the more demanding and churlish the patient becomes the more the staff will withdraw. This lack of understanding on the part of nurses will only intensify the patient's feelings of helplessness and frustration. And, in the patient with a type A personality, he will respond with overt rage or turn it into a frank depression.

The family may also be experiencing anger. The anger may be directed at the staff, the patient, or both. If the patient had been previously aware that he had certain risk factors which could lead to a heart attack, and yet he did not follow his physician's advice, the family may be very angry with him. "See what happened because you didn't give up smoking or lose weight?" And, of course, what they also mean is, "Because of your behavior you have threatened all of us, as a family, with your loss."

The patient may not be the only one to feel the family's ire. The nurses and doctors may also receive their share. Criticism of everyone from the physician to the housekeeper who cleans the room may be the tenor of the day. The complete frustration of being unable to do anything except sit and wait and suffer often seeks relief in anger.

Anger, however, is not always externalized. For this reason it is usually in this second phase of crisis that depression begins. Rathe et al. (1973) show that more than fifty percent of patients hospitalized for treatment of ischemic heart disease show moderate to severe depression. The same authors also report a direct correlation between the severity of the disease and the chronicity of the depression.

Depression is an integral part of grieving. According to the American Psychiatric Association, depressive neurosis is "manifested by an excessive reaction of depression to an internal conflict or to an identifiable event such as the loss of a love object or cherished possession" (Freedman et al., 1976, p. 634). What is more cherished than our good health?

Depression, unfortunately, assumes a myriad of forms. For cardiac patients it may evidence itself as a prolongation of chest pain without sufficient physical evidence that the patient should be having pain. Or it may present itself as apathy, lethargy, sleeping for prolonged periods of time without medication, or insomnia and agitation with sudden spells of crying. Whatever the symptoms the depressed patient expresses, he is experiencing profound feelings of betrayal and guilt. Not only has his body betrayed him but he may feel he has betrayed himself. The patient may ruminate over every aspect of his life, reminding himself of what he could or should have done. Nor will his family fail to do the same. If the spouse nagged about his smoking or eating habits she'll feel guilty because perhaps she nagged too much. If the opposite was true, then she'll feel guilty because, "I didn't make him do what he was supposed to do." Either way they both play a no win game.

Regardless of how their emotional turmoil is expressed it should be evident to the nursing staff caring for the patient and his family that the work of grieving has begun. Grief that assumes the form of anger and depression may be physiologically destructive to the patient. As indicated earlier, stress induces secretion of the catecholamines, epinephrine and norepinephrine. What has also become clear in laboratory experimentation and in autopsy studies, is that stress also induces secretion of the adrenal corticoids (Raab, 1966). The synergistic action of the adreno-corticoid-medullary response is that of severe myocardial hypoxia and electrolyte imbalance. In some cases, this response has produced diffuse subendocardial necrosis (Raab). This underlying mechanism of myocardial destruction under stress brought on by the emotional response of anger and depression can lead to a positive feedback cycle. That is, anger and depression cause increased medullary-cortical secretion, causing pain and arrythmias; which, in turn, causes increased emotional stress. Unless the nursing staff can therapeutically intervene in the emotional response, the physiologic response will continue. The ramifications of this psycho-physiologic response on a defect in an already compromised myocardium are profound: possible arrythmias, infarct extension, cardio-pulmonary de-compensation, and ultimately death.

Grieving is necessary in order to relinquish one stage of life and move into the next. But for grieving to be constructive this phase of crisis must necessarily be short. It can be shortened if the nursing staff caring for the patient do not react to the patient with the like emotion of anger but, instead, respond to his underlying grief and shock.

The mobilization of the patient and family's own internal and external resources announces the beginning of phase three. Optimally, this transition should occur while the patient is still hospitalized. Often it does not. This is a time for "picking up the pieces." The implication here is that the patient and his family have accepted the reality of heart disease and have begun to look to the future. The future may still appear bleak, but they exhibit a willingness to look at it. The family seeks the help they need to face the future together.

Now the staff who have been caring for the patient and his family may see the fruits of its labor. There is an evident willingness on the part of the patient and family to learn. The patient will usually want to know "*exactly* what happened." He wishes to know "*exactly*" what the future holds regarding wellness or illness. It is as if patient and family are seeking security in knowing all they can about their form of heart disease—hoping that in knowledge there may be safety. Hope is the predominant emotion now. "I have gone down into the valley of death and I will fear no evil."

At this stage the family seeks reassurance. Their questions center around the "how to" of getting well. The bargaining for wellness predominates. "If I follow the diet, exercise, and medication plan outlined for me will I be able to do everything I did before?" "Will I live long enough to care for my family and see them financially secure?" "If I do what you want, can you guarantee what I want?"

With questions such as these it is no wonder that those of us in the health care field are somewhat infected with the feeling of omnipotence. The patient and family now view the health care team as their saviors. A short time ago in the midst of their rage, guilt, and depression, no one could do anything right. Now, the staff can do no wrong. Placed in its proper perspective this new attitude is yet another facet of grieving. The family is desperately clinging to life and looking for the knowledge and emotional security upon which to anchor their future. During this phase the patient will need the most detailed instructions and will understand you in the most literal terms. Do not expect them to extrapolate specifics from general instructions. It is impossible for this patient and his family to theorize about the meaning of the illness or conceptualize the goals of recovery and rehabilitation. They want a cookbook program to wellness.

When I first began working as a nurse clinician with post-myocardial infarct patients and their families, it was assumed that if they were given the goals of care for the period of recovery and rehabilitation they would be able to develop their own specific guidelines. A very erroneous assumption! A short case history illustrates this point.

A 39-year-old male was admitted to the coronary care unit with a major anterolateral wall infarct. The patient was born in Berlin, Germany and had lived through the bombing of that city during the Second World War. He and his family emigrated to Canada in the late 1940s. As a young adult he came to the United States and married a girl of German descent. They had one son, who, at the time of the father's admission, was fourteen years of age. By profession, this patient was a computer programmer. By personality, he worked hard, played hard, and thoroughly enjoyed rich food,

especially butter and eggs. Although not obese, the patient
had two major risk factors prior to his M.I.: significant hyper-
cholesterolemia and chain smoking. He was definitely a type
A personality.

The week prior to discharge was spent in giving the patient
general instructions regarding the length of his recovery
period, the need for gradual increase of activities, the necessity of dietary restriction regarding saturated fats, and the
purpose of the medications he would be taking at home. The
patient and his wife appeared to understand what was being
discussed and asked good questions. The only specific instructions regarded diet and medication. The specific prescriptions were: he was not to climb stairs or go outside until
he returned for his first office appointment. The patient
asked about resuming sexual relations with his wife. It was
the cardiologist's opinion that the desire for sexual intercourse did not return until the patient felt well. So, the
patient was told that when he felt well enough he could
resume sexual relations if he assumed the passive position.
However, he was cautioned that sexual desire might not return for several weeks.

Five days later this patient was readmitted to the hospital in
congestive heart failure. Why? He and his wife had engaged in
sexual intercourse every day since his discharge from the hospital. The patient had obeyed our instructions to the letter.
His wife was following the dietary instructions in her cooking
perfectly. The patient was taking his medications according to
the prescriptions, and he was not climbing stairs. When asked
why he and his wife had relations immediately he said,
"We've been apart for three weeks! I love her and felt like
it!" The patient was then asked if he had assumed the passive
position. "Oh that, I really didn't know what you meant,
so we went ahead as we always have."

The above history graphically illustrates the need for specific, detailed instructions prior to discharge. This is not to
say that a patient and family should not be given the general

parameters of the anticipated length of time for recovery and rehabilitation, but they also need *specific, detailed, written* instructions. Writing instructions takes more time for the nurse but it helps insure that patients will have a clearer understanding of instructions and will not be under- or over-exerting themselves, especially during the first few weeks at home, which is a critical period in their recovery.

Some of you may be surprised that underexertion was mentioned. Frequently, the spouse becomes overprotective of the patient. Oversolicitousness by the spouse may not have been apparent during the patient's hospitalization. Upon re-turning home the spouse's fear that death or possible rein-farction may occur cause him or her to perform the most menial tasks for the patient, sometimes imposing a closer supervision than the patient may have received in the hos-pital (Crawshaw, 1974; Wishnie et al., 1971). The discharge of the patient from the hospital is very gratifying for the spouse but then she or he may feel the loss of the under-standing and support experienced during the patient's hospi-talization. The anxiety the spouse feels is analogous to that experienced by many patients the first few days after they leave the coronary care unit. Anxiety, an accompaniment to the grieving response, forms the basis of overprotectiveness and may only succeed in establishing a day-to-day battle-ground for control between spouse and patient. Anger and hostility build between them and often words are said and activities engaged in "just to show" the other who is boss. This emotional tug of war is most common when both spouses exhibit type A behavior.

One means of circumventing this situation is a list of written instructions that specify the do's and don'ts for a prescribed period of time. Written instructions remove the onus of having to be "boss." As one patient stated, "When-ever we are about to argue whether or not I can do a thing, we check the refrigerator door." (Discharge instructions were posted on the refrigerator door.)

The goals of recovery and rehabilitation for the patient and family with arteriosclerotic heart disease are:

1. To return them to the highest levels of wellness they are capable of attaining physiologically and psychologically.
2. To assist them in moderating their type A behavior to a more serene and less competitive level.

The attainment of these goals takes time and patience on the part of the physician, nurse, and family. The goals of care will not be accomplished in six weeks or three months. Individuals with heart disease are starting off on a lifetime of reconstructing goals and attitudes. Activities will change, relationships may alter, and ultimately some goals will be relinquished as untenable. Phase three—mobilization of resources—is the beginning of reorientation for the patient and his family. However, to remain at this state of dependence on physician and nurse, both in actuality and in feeling, would be destructive to the goal of reestablishing their own autonomy.

So far we have seen the correlation of the stages of grieving: anger-denial, depression, bargaining, resignation, with the phases of crisis: impact, turmoil, and mobilization of resources. Long-term reconstruction characterizes the fourth phase of crisis just as acceptance characterizes the fifth stage of grief. It is only when patient and family have accepted the reality of heart disease that crisis resolution through goal reconstruction can occur.

The changes and adaptations that the patient and family have undergone thus far will either prove growth-producing with an improved level of functioning, or psychological, somatic, and interpersonal disorders may become chronic (Freedman et al., 1976). Regardless of the reasoned empathetic care a patient and family have received, their modes of adaptation prior to the onset of illness will not be changed by the present crisis. Where maladaptation existed in the past these responses will only be reinforced and exaggerated in the present.

The meaning of heart disease differs for each individual and family required to cope with it. The fact that onset usually occurs in middle age is a significant variable in itself. For some patients it will mean a sanction to give up the life struggle with honor. To others it may just be another hurdle to cross in the pursuit of life's goals. For a few, heart disease may never be acknowledged as more than a passing problem. "I'll wear out, not rust out."

Patients in whom depression deepens and becomes a chronic debilitating state turn from being physically and mentally capable individuals into invalids. Their act of giving up exemplifies their feeling of total loss. Verbally or behaviorally they make the statement of wishing to die. Patients in this state of mind should be given a psychiatric referral, either to a master's prepared psychiatric–mental health nurse or to a psychiatrist.

The question is asked: How does a nonpsychiatric nurse or physician determine when an emotional maladaptive response is present? Answer: when depression is the prime cause of an individual's inability to resume his place in society as a contributing member. How do you know that depression may be the causative factor? Answer: when the patient's physiological parameters are returning to normal or near normal levels but his emotional response is not. As recovery progresses, the patient's feeling of well-being should correspond to the physiologic indications of return to health. The nurse should assess the patient's nonverbal behaviors as well as listen to his statements. For instance, excessive sleeping, spontaneous crying without provocation, and lack of appetite are some indicators of increasing depression. The symptomatology of depression in other patients may include insomnia, agitation, and chronic constipation. Careful questioning on the part of the nurse will usually elicit from the patient the admission to feeling blue, hopeless, and preoccupied with his somatic symptoms (Freedman et al., 1976). In fact, some patients hide their depression so well that their preoccupation with somatic complaints which cannot be verified upon physical examination may be the nurse or physician's only clue as to the patient's actual state of mind.

A woman in her early forties was admitted to the hospital following a cardiovascular accident (CVA) secondary to rheumatic heart disease. The primary diagnosis was mitral stenosis with atrial fibrillation which developed following adult onset of rheumatic fever. She was a wife and mother of several children ranging in age from late teens to eight-year-old twins. Until her illness, she had been an active member of her community. The CVA was considered mild and it was anticipated that she would fully recover with only minimal left sided weakness. During hospitalization her physical improvement proceeded rapidly. The patient was emotionally labile, but this was dismissed by the physician as a post CVA syndrome. The patient was receptive to predischarge planning and teaching and appeared to understand that with short-term physical therapy she would regain full use of her left arm and leg. By the time of discharge the patient was walking well and was regaining fine control of finger movements of her left hand.

A few days following the patient's discharge from the hospital, I made a visit to her home and was greeted at the door by a friend of the family. The patient was in bed although she had been encouraged to be up and move about as much as possible. Upon arriving home from the hospital she took to her bed and refused to get up even for meals. Physical examination revealed good function on the affected side and no change in her cardiac status. The patient stated she felt blue and couldn't keep from crying. The physician was contacted and ordered the tranquilizer Librium, rather than an antidepressant. By the end of the second week the patient's depression deepened, she became agitated and attempted to take all the Librium ordered. After repeated attempts to obtain a psychiatric referral through the patient's attending physician, I made a direct referral to a psychiatrist known to her. The patient was seen the next morning. Within a matter of three weeks the patient's depression moderated to the extent that she again was taking an interest in her husband, children, and limited outside activity. Now her physical and emotional health allowed the patient to re-establish a satisfactory equilibrium in her life.

Some patients unfortunately do not receive the benefits of psychiatric intervention. Treating the symptoms of anxiety and depression as if these are manifestations of cardiac pathology tends to prolong the patient's disability. In some cases, it may render that disability permanent.

REDIRECTION OF LIFE GOALS

The act of grieving over the loss of the patient's previous state of health is essentially completed when the patient and his family feel free to plan for the future. Life style or life goals may be altered or remain unchanged. The family now considers the alternatives available to them in achieving these goals.

For some families a radical change in life style may be required, but they now have the capacity to plan how that change will occur. Some relinquished goals are replaced by others more realistically attainable. Major or minor adaptations are made according to the family's basic decision regarding the quantity and quality of life desired. Sir William Osler is said to have remarked that one of the best ways of assuring a long life is to suffer a mild heart attack in middle age. A man may now feel that he has sufficient reason to cease driving himself and enjoy leisure activities, and to give more of his time to family and friends.

The excuse of a heart attack may also serve as a psychological crutch. Whatever the reasons an individual may choose to rely on it, the prop of ill health should not be removed unless something perceived as more valuable by the patient replaces it (Lidz, 1968). On the other hand, we have already seen the devastating effects of oversolicitousness on a patient's emotional state.

The role of the nurse and physician is now to advise, suggest, and guide. Future health care decisions are now the prerogative of the family. For the patient and family the crisis is over, grieving essentially is completed, and life must go on. The patient experiences an intense joie de vivre and elan vital. Life is very precious after one experiences and accepts his own mortality.

REFERENCES

Caplan, G. 1964. *Principles of preventive psychiatry.* New York: Basic Books, Inc.

Crawshaw, J. E. 1974. Community rehabilitation after acute M.I. *Heart and Lung* 3:258.

Freedman, A. M.; Kaplan, H. I.; and Sadock, B. J. 1976. *Modern synopsis of a comprehensive textbook of psychiatry, Volume 2.* 2nd ed. Baltimore: Williams and Wilkins Company.

Glass, D. C. 1976. Stress, competition and heart attacks. *Psychology Today* 134:54–58.

Jenkins, C. D. 1971. Psychological and social precursors of coronary disease. *New England Journal of Medicine* 284:244–307.

Jenkins, C. D.; Roseman, R. H.; and Zyzanski, S. J. 1974. Prediction of clinical coronary heart disease by a test for the coronary prone behavior pattern. *New England Journal of Medicine* 290:1271.

Kubler-Ross, E. 1969. *On death and dying.* New York: Macmillan Company.

Langsley, D., and Kaplan, D. 1968. *The treatment of families in crisis.* New York: Grune and Stratton.

Lidz, T. 1968. *The person: his development throughout the life cycle.* New York: Basic Books, Inc.

Moriyama, I. M.; Kruegar, D. E.; and Stamler, J. 1971. *Cardiovascular disease in the United States.* Cambridge, Mass.: Harvard University Press.

Moss, A. J.; Wynar, B.; and Goldstein, S. 1969. Delay in hospitalization during the acute coronary period. *American Journal of Cardiology* 24:659.

Raab, W. 1966. Emotional and sensory stress factors in myocardial pathology. *American Heart Journal* 4:539–56.

Rathe, R. H.; Tuffi, C. F.; Suchor, R. J.; and Arthur, R. J. 1973. Group therapy in the outpatient management of postmyocardial infarction patients. *Psychiatric Medicine* 4:77.

Tibblin, G.; Lindstrom, B.; and Ander, S. 1972. Emotions and heart disease. *Ciba Foundation Symposium* 8:321.

Wishnie, H. A.; Hackett, T. P.; and Cassem, N. H. 1971. Psychological hazards of convalescence following M.I. *JAMA* 215:1292.

ADDITIONAL BIBLIOGRAPHY

Gentry, D. W., and Williams, R. B., Jr. 1975. *Psychological aspects of myocardial infarction and coronary care.* St. Louis: C. V. Mosby Company.

Greyton, A. G. 1976. *Textbook of medical psychology.* Philadelphia: W. B. Saunders Company.

Halberstam, M., and Lesher, S. 1976. *A coronary event.* Philadelphia: J. B. Lippincott Company.

Hellerstein, H. K., and Freedman, A. M. 1970. Sexual activity and the postcoronary patient. *Archives of Internal Medicine* 125:987–99.

Kimball, P. C. 1970. Conceptual development in psychosomatic medicine: 1939–1969. *Annals of Internal Medicine* 73:307–16.

Lynch, J. J. 1977. *The broken heart: the medical consequences of loneliness.* New York: Basic Books, Inc.

Menninger, K. 1938. *Man against himself.* New York: Harcourt, Brace and World, Inc.

Naughton, J. P., and Hellerstein, H. K. 1973. *Exercise testing and exercise testing in coronary heart disease.* New York: Academic Press.

Podell, R. N.; Kent, D.; and Keller, K. 1976. Patient psychological defenses and physician responses in the long-term treatment of hypertension. *Journal of Family Practice* 3:145–49.

Scalzi, C. C. 1973. Nursing management of behavioral responses following an acute myocardial infarction. *Heart and Lung* 2:62–69.

Seligman, M. E. P. 1974. Submissive death: giving up on life. *Psychology Today,* May, 80–85.

Shepard, R. S. 1971. *Human physiology.* Philadelphia: J. B. Lippincott Company.

Stockwell, M. L. 1968. Depression: an operational definition with themes related to nursing role. In *Developing behavioral concepts in nursing,* ed. L. Zulroa and H. C. Belcher. Atlanta, Georgia: Southern Region Education Board.

CHAPTER FIVE

Grief in Parents of a Child with a Birth Handicap

Ann M. Zuzich

INTRODUCTION

Much has been written about the family system reorientation that must take place when a new member enters the family and the disruption in family life that occurs at the transition into parenthood (Dyer, 1963; LeMasters, 1957; Rossi, 1975).

When the infant is handicapped, there are additional variables that affect the nature of the relationships with the parents and siblings. Although it is questionable that all families experiencing such an event are thrown into an emotional crisis (Begab, 1964; Farber, 1964), it is generally believed that most families experience some degree of grief.

The literature reveals statements from parents demonstrating their intense feeling of grief. One parent wrote her response to the physician who informed her of her child's disability:

I sat staring at him unable to voice intelligent response. No physical pain ever compared to this. With a fist resting gravely against his chin, he sat waiting to answer any questions I might have. But the shock left no room for questions. I felt only grief. No one could erase the facts. The words kept playing back in my ears, "brain damage," not weeks, not months, years! (St. Cyr, 1970, p. 31).

Several days after the birth of his first child, a victim of Down's Syndrome, a father described his feelings by saying, "I feel like I'm in mourning. I feel that I should not be dressed this way (in business suit) . . . that I should be wearing a black suit. . . . I feel that I'm in mourning" (Hart, 1970, p. 59).

THE GRIEF SYNDROME

Studies have identified acute grief as a definite syndrome with psychological and somatic symptomatology (Lindemann, 1965; Caplan, 1964). Lindemann lists five points pathognomic for grief: (1) somatic distress; (2) preoccupation with the image of the deceased; (3) guilt; (4) hostile reactions; and (5) loss of patterns of conduct (p. 10). These responses are often identified in family members where there is a handicapped child. Lindemann further explains that it must be understood that grief reactions are just one form of separation reaction. Separation may occur from causes other than death. In the instance of the birth of a handicapped child, it is proposed that the final and irreversible separation precipitating the grief response is separation from the fantasy, a formulation proposed by Kroman (1977). One father has referred to this in writing of the myths perpetrated by society, which promote many problems for parents of handicapped children. Among these, often wholly believed by the young, are the notions that marriage is a state of "eternal bliss" and that out of this "blissful union" come children who are physically and mentally beautiful and perfect (Grier, 1977, p. 23). Parents who view their children as sources of vicarious satisfaction are particularly vulnerable to this "fantasy" separation in their overwhelming realization that this handicapped child will not excel physically, intellectually, or financially. Most parents have great anticipations about their babies. Solnit and Stark (1961) have stated that parents often expect a perfect child, not merely a typical one.

Particularly significant is the fact that the opportunity for the successful accomplishment of the "grief work" in response to the fantasy loss is very limited, if it exists at all. Lindemann believes that the duration of the grief reaction depends upon the success with which the "grief work" is performed, "that is, achieves emancipation from the bondage to the deceased, readjustment to the environment in which the deceased is missing and the formation of new relationships" (1965, pp. 10–11). He found that the greatest obstacle to this work seemed to be the avoidance of the discomfort associated with the grief experience and the necessary emotional response. One mother of a mentally handicapped child wrote:

> Pages could be written on this one thing—the psychological impact on the parents of having a grief which they cannot unburden because of the pressure of public opinion . . . this aspect can cause more real suffering and wreak more real havoc to the personalities involved than the mental retardation itself (Murray, 1956, p. 64).

Olshansky (1963) proposed his concept of "chronic sorrow" based on this inability to internalize the sorrow that is felt along with the factors in our society that place the child and his family in the devalued segment of our society.

Coupled with the perception of a limited number of people to whom the parent can openly express grief over the fantasy loss are the demands of immediately responding to the multiple needs of a handicapped infant. "If the bereavement occurs at a time when the patient is confronted with important tasks and when there is necessity for maintaining the morale of others, he may show little or no reaction for weeks or even much longer" (Lindemann, p. 13). Thus, the grief work is often delayed—often for years—with resulting maladaptive behaviors, many of which were identified by Lindemann. For example, severe reactions to separations were found to have their source in earlier, unresolved grief reactions. In addition, unexplainable somatic responses, specific medical diseases such as ulcerative colitis, and altered relationships with friends, relatives, and others, were all associated with unresolved grief. Practitioners have repeatedly reported the occurrence of these same reactions in parents after the birth of a handicapped child.

Schroeder (1974) reported on a study of twelve families who experienced the birth of a handicapped child where all of the stages of the grief process as delineated by Lindemann (1965) and categorized by Engel (1964) were found. Schroeder also found that the grieving process in these families seemed "more ongoing than when related to death." Since the ages of the handicapped children ranged from one month to ten years and the interview segments that Schroeder reported indicated little support for parents to engage at the appropriate time in grief work, it is easy to suspect that the ongoing nature of the grieving process was predictable as an outcome of delayed or omitted grief work (p. 162).

COPING WITH THE CRISIS OF A HANDICAPPED CHILD

The potential for family crisis that the birth of the handicapped child presents is often realized. Using the field-oriented model of crisis theory as presented by Langsley and Kaplan (1968), it is easy to understand why the development of a crisis is almost inevitable in families where there is the birth of a handicapped child. Identifying the work of Lindemann and Caplan as a stress-oriented model, Langsley and Kaplan expand the model by postulating that the outcome and the existence of a crisis may depend on the social field. This framework is particularly applicable where the stressful event is the birth of a handicapped child, a circumstance that is heavily loaded in our society by conflicting attitudes and values which are reflected in the literature (President's Committee on Mental Retardation, 1975; Fletcher, 1972). These conflicts have affected the ability of the established systems of the society to respond to the needs of the handicapped, who are alternately viewed as devalued human beings, or as saints. It is suggested that such a social field will, indeed, be a contributing factor in the development of a crisis situation at the birth of a handicapped child.

Ordinary coping methods are doomed to failure, thereby precipitating a crisis as the parent faces either alternative. One young mother who had just been informed that her newborn was multiply handicapped was being consoled by a clergyman, who said, "You must remember that you are the mother of a saint!" She cried out, in reply, "I don't want to be the mother of a saint, I want to be the mother of a normal baby!" Ready to accept the role of a mother of a normal baby, she was unprepared to cope with the role of mother of a saint, and the stage was set for crisis.

The role of devalued human being, or even nonperson, which is ascribed by society to handicapped individuals is particularly conducive to the precipitation of crisis when a handicapped child is born. Not only was the parent prepared to accept the role of parent of a normal child, but the ascribed role of the offspring now carries with it the devaluation of the parent, as well as the implication that such a parent is a threat to the well-being of society in significant ways. If there are genetic causes for the handicap, a justification for the exercise of the procreative function is demanded and the implications of procreation for such parents because of the impact on the genetic pool is widely debated.

In the absence of genetic causes, the parent faces the dilemma of either accepting the role of devalued member of society along with the handicapped child, rejecting the de-valued child, or assuming the role of advocate for all handi-capped, devalued persons. In any case, crisis is inevitable until the parents are able to resolve the dilemma created by the social field within which the event occurs.

Menolascino identifies "novelty shock" as an immediate response of families to the birth of a mentally handicapped child (1977, p. 244). Parents have written of this response. St. Cyr wrote of her shock and grief as she left the physician's office where she had just been told that her baby was brain-damaged.

> I wanted most to be alone. Oblivious of the few pas-sengers, but fully aware of the several empty seats, I walked pensively to the rear of the coach where I was least likely to be intruded upon (1970, pp. 31–32).

Schroeder reported that mothers most often expressed the question, "Why? Why me?" One mother in her study spoke of her disbelief. She said, "It's just always something that happens to somebody else, like an accident or something like that. You can't really believe it's happened" (1974, p. 162).

Menolascino reports that the intensity of the novelty shock response is often not related to the reality of the handicap. Equally intense responses have been reported for widely differing degrees of handicapping conditions (1977, p. 244).

Many times the parents know nothing about the condition that is affecting the child. Inability to understand the ter-minology leads to erroneous decision making that may have lifelong impact. For example, I encountered one mother who was in treatment for an emotional illness and was not making significant progress toward recovery. Her husband reported to a nurse friend that her illness began, he believed, three years before, after the birth of their little girl with Down's

Syndrome. It was their fourth child. At the time, the father was advised to place the child in an institution immediately so that the mother would not "develop a relationship with her" and to help the mother to understand that it would be inadvisable for her to see her "deformed baby." He willingly followed this advice and the mother left the hospital without the baby. The mother had never seen the child, even though the little girl was residing in a state agency not far from the family's home. The father had not seen the child since her birth, when he was informed of her condition. Furthermore, there was a taboo on any discussion of the child in the family since such discussion might produce unhappiness and serious discomfort in the parents. The father confessed to lack of knowledge of the term, Down's Syndrome; he believed that the child would die "probably in five years or so," and that she would never be able to walk or talk. He said that his wife had not been able to discuss this event with her therapist, and he wondered if this child's birth was related to his wife's present mental illness. These parents were eventually reunited with their baby with resultant relief of the mother's symptomatology.

Furthermore, the state of shock and disbelief does not allow some parents to receive information about the child's condition. Nurses, physicians, and other health care providers need to be particularly sensitive to the degree of shock that is being experienced by the parents. The bewilderment, confusion, and disorganization that result are not apt to promote attentiveness and receptivity to information. The provision of understanding support accompanied by the selection of the appropriate time is essential if the parents are to be helped to receive factual knowledge; always, repetition of essential facts is necessary, with the parents being actively encouraged to ask for further clarification.

The significance of the family's perception of the event is crucial. Effective assistance will be immediate and will include assistance in perceiving the reality. Such assistance can only come from professionals who are well informed and who have honestly sought to clarify their own values related to the birth of handicapped children.

Aguilera and Messick (1978) have presented a paradigm for crisis intervention that is useful in understanding the effect of balancing factors in the presence of a stressful event. (See Figure 1.) Realistic perception is vital in the reacquisition of emotional equilibrium that may be disturbed by a stressful event. When there is distorted perception there is no relationship between the event and the feelings of stress. Realistic perception can be promoted by the attitudes and knowledge of the persons in the environment, particularly physicians, nurses, and significant family members. While not diminishing the seriousness of the condition, factual knowledge and assistance in problem solving should be provided, using all available resources.

SITUATIONAL SUPPORTS

Another balancing factor identified in the paradigm is adequate situational support. Situational supports mean those persons who are in the environment who can be relied upon to help solve the stressful problem. Menolascino (1977) speaks of reality stress that results from the situational support to include easy availability of concrete and direct services. Such services should be immediately available when the handicapped child is born. Recent approaches to assisting mentally and physically handicapped persons to move toward self-fulfillment have provided new hope for such persons and their families, but the success of these approaches can be significantly diminished through delay in planning. Input from professionals representing many disciplines constitutes a transdisciplinary effort that is essential for effective impact. Implementation of the transdisciplinary model of care demands that nurses and physicians present at the birth be

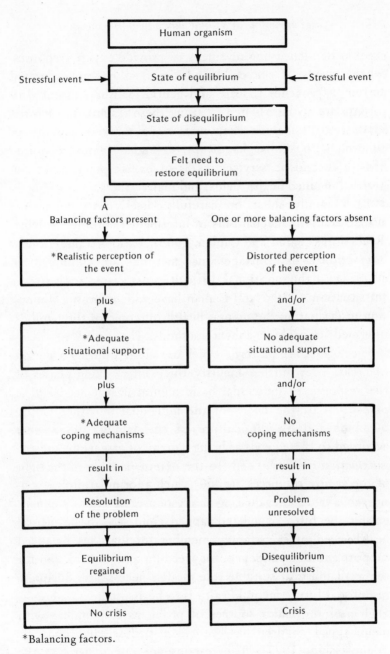

*Balancing factors.

FIGURE 1. Effect of Balancing Factors in a Stressful Event

From Aguilera, D. C., and Messick, J. M. 1978. *Crisis intervention: theory and methodology*. Saint Louis: C. V. Mosby Company. p. 68.

capable of identifying resources to provide expert responses to the needs of the child and the family. Knowledge of current approaches to care and gentle realism is essential if parents are to be assisted in using these resources. Such resources might include clergymen, social workers, parents of children with similar handicaps, extended family, comprehensive diagnostic services, skills of expert practitioners in health and allied health fields, and many others.

Each family must be carefully assessed to determine available coping mechanisms or intermediate problem-solving mechanisms (Parad and Caplan, 1965). Various transactional, interactional, and intrapersonal methods are employed in adapting to the emotional difficulties associated with stressful situations. Parad and Caplan have added another dimension in evaluating the mental health outcome of the family's intermediate problem-solving methods. They speak of assessing need-response patterns which are altered during a period of crisis. They further identify three interlocking phases of the response to individual basic mental health needs: "the *perception* of the needs of the individual by other family members and by the culture of the family, the *respect* accorded to these needs as being worthy of attention, and the *satisfaction* of these needs to the extent possible in the light of the family resources" (p. 60). Such a formulation has considerable value in evaluating the responses of a family experiencing the birth of a handicapped child. The basic mental health need of each family member for love, for balanced support and independence, for freedom and control, and for the availability of suitable role models necessitates adequate response if future mental health is to be assured.

One of the major sources of problems for families with handicapped children has been identified as value conflicts (Menolascino, 1977). The response of our society to the deviant or marginally deviant individual has generally been to attach a negative value to him. Parents are often caught in severe inner conflict because of this. Menolascino has provided a diagrammatic approach to exploring and meeting the family management needs of parents of the retarded in which he includes management of value conflicts as a part of the third stage of a sequence of responses (1970, p. 487). Suggested intervention includes the concepts already presented with emphasis on prevention of the family disintegration and dysfunction characteristic of crisis situations. Since the birth of the handicapped child will precipitate a grief response in the family, encouragement and support must be provided for the necessary grief to take place.

Schumann (1974) has provided some guidelines for hospital nurses giving this kind of assistance to the mother.

1. Sit down as close as possible to the mother and try to look relaxed and unhurried.
2. Establish eye contact.
3. Introduce yourself by name and job classification.
4. State gently and clearly that you are sorry this tragedy has happened to her.
5. If this starts her crying, as it usually does, put your arms around her and encourage her to do so.
6. In the meantime, you can assess some of her needs and mentally formulate a tentative plan of nursing care for meeting them (p. 48).

This intervention should be extended to include the father and the siblings. It is wise to assist the father to understand that the grieving process is acceptable and even advisable, and that the nurse is willing and able to share his grief. Children in the family need to have honest explanations and the opportunity to share in the grieving process. Many parents have difficulty in being truthful with their nonhandicapped children, thus setting the scene for fantasies and unnecessary fears. Nurses, physicians, and others can help parents by encouraging them to include the children in any discussion with the professionals beginning immediately in the hospital, if possible. Such discussions should continue in the home after mother and baby are discharged; the public health nurse or the visiting nurse can make an important contribution here. Not only can the nurse provide the necessary supportive presence for the grief work of the family to take place, he or she can also provide for the care of the handicapped child permitting the mother to attend to the grieving process. Peretz (1970) has reported the duration of the acute phase of the normal grief response to be one to two months. It has been suggested that the feeling of grief following the birth of a handicapped child is considerably longer than that. The minimum expectation is that the intense grief will be experienced for the period of time described by Peretz (p. 22).

It is important to remember that the birth of a handicapped child results in a state of shock; the resulting confusion and bewilderment can be alleviated by the attending care providers. It is at this point that professionals can be of great assistance in helping the family perceive the entire event in a realistic way. Such assistance must begin immediately in hospitals where the parents begin to sort out the confusion that most of them report. This demands that the professional assist the parents in acquiring immediate access to someone who can speak with them about the current approaches to care. Nothing can be so devastating to the parent of a child with Down's Syndrome, for instance, or to the child himself, than to be advised that the baby should be immediately placed in an institution or other alternative living situation, with the unspoken message that the tragedy of the child's birth is overwhelming and that nothing can be done. Such messages from professional caregivers reflect abysmal ignorance on the professional's part and unforgivable negligence in not seeking out someone who can assist parents to realistically perceive this event in their lives. At the very least, parents should be helped to meet with other parents of children with similar handicapping conditions. The local unit of the Association for Retarded Citizens, the Spina Bifida

Association, and other parent groups are available in most major cities in the United States to respond to this kind of need. In the event that the infant's physical condition remains serious, or even critical, professionals must be available to assist the parents through the grief process. Little is accomplished—and, in fact, harm is done—when the parents are encouraged to avoid such necessary involvement. The mother of the child with an encephalocele wrote that when she was finally permitted to hold her child,

> At that moment nothing else mattered, there were no thoughts of encephaloceles or life spans, only that we were finally able to cuddle and be close, just as any mother and baby should (Donnelly, 1974, p. 51).

Later, after the baby's death at three weeks of age, this same mother wrote,

> I was luckier than many mothers of defective babies, my baby lived three weeks and I had an opportunity to get to know her. How could I face myself now if I had followed the doctor's advice that I dissociate myself from her? Perhaps those who tried to protect me from facing reality thought the experience of the pregnancy and the birth could be erased by choice and by avoiding the child (Donnelly, 1974, p. 51).

The long-term detrimental effect of contributing through ignorance and incompetence to the novelty shock that the parents are experiencing has been observed by many practitioners in this field. "If we fail at this point to help parents understand their child's problems, we may well be sending them further along the path of carousel medicine, or what has been termed shopping patterns for further diagnostic services, rather than affective treatment intervention" (Menolascino, 1977, p. 244). In addition to information and factual knowledge, it is necessary to be certain that caution be used in making predictions. Particularly offensive is the prediction, "Your child will die before the age of two—or five— or. . . ." I have repeatedly encountered tragic situations that have evolved because families accepted such a prediction, building lifetime plans around it. Surely the professional must accept that such predictions have little validity. One mother reported her own experiences,

> Well . . . the initial reaction, I would say took a good six to nine months to get over. Mainly as I said, it goes back to them telling me he wouldn't live. If they hadn't done that, I can look back and see that our whole lives would have been different. Because every time that baby would sneeze, I'd rush him to the emergency room. "Oh, he's dying now—they told me he wasn't going to live!" I just sat and held him all the time. I had two other kids, let's see at that time they would have been like—oh—three and five. And I just neglected them completely and neglected my husband, my home, everything. I'd get up in the morning and sit and rock him all day, and if nothing got done—well fine! Because they told me he wasn't going to live, and I was going to spend every minute with him (Schroeder, 1974, p. 165).

Recognizing that the birth of a handicapped child is anxiety provoking for both the professional and the family, it is not unreasonable to expect the professional to be able to cope with his/her anxiety in less destructive ways.

VALUE REORIENTATION

It has been recognized that a necessary value reorganization takes place in families where there is a successful integration of the handicapped child into the family. Such a value reorientation must also take place among the professionals whose work involves contact with these families. At the least, professionals must make attempts to clarify their own values, so that the messages communicated to families are clear. Such value clarification is not easy or comfortable. Questions to be addressed might include:

1. Do you believe that the infant with a severe handicap at birth has the right to live?
2. If that right does not exist, what are the criteria by which the decision is made to support life in one case and not in another?
3. Do you believe that the care of handicapped children is a responsibility of society?
4. Do you believe in the concept of equal right to health care, to education, to adequate housing regardless of the degree of handicapping condition?

Persons who are available for situational support are of great significance in assisting families. Their behavior will reflect the values that they hold. In the early confusion and bewilderment that parents experience, the behavior of the persons around them is of great importance in assisting them to shape their own responses. When handicapped persons are encountered whose families have rejected them, it is tempting to wonder how much assistance the family had from the "helping professionals" to assume their rejecting posture. The value of group discussions to resolve value conflict and to reorient has been demonstrated. It would be relatively easy to institute this mechanism among the personnel on hospital staffs. Many hospitals have clergymen available whose participation in such a group could be very helpful. The group discussion for care providers could also be implemented in public health agencies, schools, and other agencies whose personnel inevitably encounter handicapped persons.

SUMMARY

The grief in parents of a child with a birth handicap is easily reactivated throughout the life of the family. It has been suggested that encouragement for the grieving process to take place at the time of the feeling of intense loss of the fantasied perfect child might alleviate intense responses at a later time. It must be admitted, however, that there is a need for research in this area. The precipitation of the crisis which any sudden loss entails must be considered as a significant part of the professional evaluation at the birth of a handicapped child. Whether that crisis occurs and whether its resolution results in a restoration of function that is on a higher level than that of the pre crisis state will depend upon the success of the methods employed to resolve the crisis. The skill and knowledge of the professional practitioners who are present and the response of society to the handicapped person are critical factors.

REFERENCES

Aguilera, D. C., and Messick, J. M. 1978. *Crisis intervention: theory and methodology.* 3rd ed. Saint Louis: C. V. Mosby Company.

Begab, M. J. 1964. The mentally retarded and the family. In *Prevention and treatment of mental retardation,* edited by I. Phillips. New York: Basic Books, Inc.

Caplan, G. 1964. *Principles of preventive psychiatry.* New York: Basic Books, Inc.

Donnelly, E. 1974. The real of her. *Journal of Gerontological Nursing* 3:48–52.

Dyer, E. D. 1963. Parenthood in crisis: a re-study. *Marriage and Family Living* 25:196–201.

Engel, G. L. 1964. Grief and grieving. *American Journal of Nursing* 9:93.

Farber, B. 1964. *Family.* San Francisco: Chandler Publishing Company.

Fletcher, J. 1972. Indication of humanhood. Hastings Center Report, no. 2, November, 1–4.

Grier, B. G. 1977. On being a parent of a handicapped child. In *Mental retardation,* eds. C. J. Drew, J. Clifford, M. L. Hardman, and H. P. Blum. Saint Louis: C. V. Mosby Company.

Hart, N. W. 1970. Frequently expressed feelings and reactions of parents toward their retarded children. In *Diminished people,* ed. N. R. Bernstein. Boston: Little, Brown and Company.

Kroman, E. 1977. Families in loss. A conference co-sponsored by the Michigan Nurses Association and the Michigan Public Health Association, 12 May 1977, Dearborn, Michigan.

Langsley, D. C., and Kaplan, D. M. 1968. *The treatment of families in crisis.* New York: Grune and Stratton.

LeMasters, E. E. 1957. Parenthood in crisis. *Marriage and Family Living* 19:352–55.

Lindemann, E. 1965. Symptomatology and management of acute grief. In *Crisis intervention: selected readings,* ed. H. J. Parad. New York: Family Service Association of America.

Menolascino, F. J. 1977. *Challenges in mental retardation.* New York: Human Sciences Press.

Menolascino, F. J. 1970. *Psychiatric approaches to mental retardation.* New York: Basic Books, Inc.

Murray, D. G. 1956. *This is Steve's story.* Nashville, Tenn.: Abingdon Press.

Olshanksky, S. 1963. Chronic sorrow: a response to having a mentally defective child. *Social Casework* 43:190–93.

Parad, H. J., and Caplan, G. 1965. A framework for studying families in crisis. In *Crisis intervention: selected readings,* ed. H. J. Parad. New York: Family Service Association of America.

Peretz, D. 1970. Reaction to loss. In *Loss and grief: psychological management in medical practice,* eds. B. Schoenberg, A. C. Carr, D. Peretz, and A. H. Kutscher. New York: Columbia University Press.

Rossi, A. S. 1975. Transition to parenthood. In *Human life cycle,* ed. C. W. Sze. New York: Jason Aronson, Inc.

Schroeder, E. 1974. The birth of a defective child: a cause for grieving. In *Nursing of families in crisis,* eds. B. P. Weaver and J. E. Hall. Philadelphia: J. B. Lippincott Company.

Schumann, H. 1974. Introduction. In E. Donnelly. The real of her. *Journal of Gerontological Nursing* 3:48–52.

Solnit, A. J., and Stark, M. H. 1961. Mourning the birth of a defective child. In *The psychoanalytic study of the child, volume 16,* eds. R. S. Eissler, H. Hartmann, A. Freud, and M. Kris. New York: International Universities Press.

St. Cyr, M. 1970. *The story of Pat.* Paramus, NJ: Paulist Press.

ADDITIONAL BIBLIOGRAPHY

Eaton, W. J., and Weil, R. J. 1955. *Culture and mental disorders: a comparative study of Hutterites and other populations.* Glencoe, IL: Free Press.

Grossman, F. K. 1977. Brothers and sisters of retarded children. In *Mental retardation,* eds. C. J. Drew, M. L. Hardman, and H. P. Blum. Saint Louis: C. V. Mosby Company.

Solomons, G. 1970. Counseling parents of the retarded: the interpretation interview. In *Psychiatric approaches to mental retardation,* ed. F. J. Menolascino. New York: Basic Books, Inc.

Zuk, G. H. et al. 1961. Maternal acceptance of retarded children: a questionnaire study of attitudes and religious background. *Child Development* 32:525–40.

CHAPTER SIX

Grief and the Process of Aging

Judith M. Agee

INTRODUCTION

Old age or aging can be examined from a number of different aspects. It can be looked at as a disease, as the ultimate tragedy, as a moral failure, or as a developmental phase. I prefer to view aging as a phase of human development. It is one phase of life that is, unfortunately, characterized by loss: social, physical, and psychological. These losses and the individual's adjustment to them comprise the basic focus of this chapter.

It is hoped that by increasing the understanding of the social and cultural status of the aging, as well as the individual's reaction to this process, the health care provider will be better able to assess the emotional needs of the elderly person and constructively plan care for him and for his family. This chapter will not deal with the physiological aspects of aging nor with physical or medical management skills although these involve an important aspect of care of the elderly. The emphasis here will be the individual's emotional reaction to his physical and psychological losses or disabilities and the implications therein for nursing care.

Those people who view the aged as either worthless, infantalized remnants, or, as difficult, angry, embittered obligations or burdens have accepted the cultural stereotypes of aging that are essentially negative. It is no wonder that the care of the elderly in the health professions is not a popular area. Even more unfortunate is the fact that these negative stereotypes of aging are often held by some aged individuals themselves. These negative stereotypes, which focus only on the debilitative aspects of the aging process and the untoward reactions of old persons to the aging process, often serve to obscure the reality of those who live a relatively happy, adaptive, and active old age.

It is not difficult to bring to mind many persons who made or are making great cultural, scientific, or professional contributions well into their seventies and eighties, such as: Arthur Rubinstein, Arturo Toscanini, Pablo Picasso, Pablo Casals, Leopold Stokowski, Arthur Fiedler, and Margaret Mead, to name a few. We often fail to recognize the chronological age of those who make contributions to our culture and are well known. To us they may appear ageless. When witness to physical endurance or accomplishments of aged friends, family, or acquaintances, we regard them as "different," "amazing," or "unusual." In other words, they do not fit our stereotype of the aged as essentially incompetent, bungling, debilitated byproducts of our society.

THE WELL-ADJUSTED ELDERLY

The literature does reflect upon the questions of patterns of aging and upon those who age with an adequate degree of gratification and morale. Perhaps it would be helpful, at this point, to examine the factors that appear to promote satisfactory adjustment to the losses, loneliness, and deprivations of aging so that these people do not appear quite so amazing or unique.

Goldfarb (1974) describes the well-adjusted elderly person as one who has retained the ability to experience gratification and meet needs. This, he states, enables the elderly person to maintain a relatively positive self-esteem, a sense of confidence, social meaningfulness, identity, and purpose in spite of the inevitable losses that occur with the aging process. The older individual who is seen as aging "well," is fortunate in three main areas seen as influential in the healthy adaptation of people: social environment, inherent biological make-up, and physical environment.

Goldfarb perceives the elderly who age successfully as having, or continuing to have, needs and drives similar to those of younger people: primarily, the needs for useful work activity and gratifying relationships. The elderly may meet these needs somewhat differently, however. For example, the aged individual may experience a warm rush of pride or heightened sense of esteem from a period of reminiscing or review of an aspect of his life rather than from present achievement or performance. Interestingly, Goldfarb's defined population of well-adjusted aged usually live in their own homes. This, in itself, often promotes a sense of pride, achievement, and dignity: in short, high morale. Heightened morale, which includes a sense of courage, enthusiasm, and confidence, appears to be a significant factor in how anyone adjusts to critical life stages.

Goldfarb identifies multiple factors that may favor, if not guarantee, high morale in the aged. Such factors as economic security, high educational level, high social status, and good health would obviously enhance the opportunities for need fulfillment, development of social contacts, coping skills, and interests. In short, good adjustment to old age appears to be closely linked to good physical and mental health coupled with favorable socioeconomic circumstances. On the other hand, deprivations complicate adequate adjustment to old age and may result in any number of physical and emotional maladjustments (1974, pp. 823–25).

AGING, GRIEVING, AND STEREOTYPES

For some of those who do not find gratifications, dignity, and heightened morale in later life, to age is to grieve. For them, to begin to think about the process of aging is to begin to grieve for the many anticipated losses that are in the offing. Many of these losses involve the giving up of manifestations of independent functioning so necessary to the preservation of self-esteem. Curtain (1972) has summarized the essence of these losses in her powerful, yet poignant statement on aging, *Nobody Ever Died of Old Age: In Praise of Old People—In Outrage at their Loneliness.*

The shrinking of the elderly person's world is accomplished through the loss of family and friends, diminishing energy apparent in the execution of even the simplest activity, the loss of gratification derived from as much food and sleep as they previously needed, the loss of human contact, and, finally, the anticipated loss of even the last remnants of independent functioning.

The major themes in the current literature related to old age are loss, dependency, helplessness, physical disability, loneliness, and depression. Palmore (1973) identifies the many social-psychological stressors of old age as diminished income, loss of social role and status, bereavement, isolation through physical or mental disability, and loss of mental or thought processes. Add to this the obvious losses of physical ability and one is left with a grim impression of aging, at best (pp. 46-47).

One could question, however, just how many of the losses of the aged are actual or are perceived as stereotypes of the aging process by others. Silverstone and Hyman (1976) contend that some of the common stereotypes of the aged person as useless, poor, and lonely are not necessarily as universally present as is thought. Many other authors challenge the stereotypes that the aged are rigid, asexual, and have lost interest in life. Kahn et al. (1975) report that complaints of memory loss are not congruent with the tested intellectual functioning of the individuals in their study. They feel that the complaint of memory loss is due more to depression than to impaired brain functioning, and they challenge the stereotype of the aged experiencing an anticipated intellectual decline (pp. 1569–73).

If these are some of the stereotypes of the aged, then what are the actualities? As has been previously mentioned, not all individuals grow old in a state of perpetual misery and anguish. On the other hand, people do not enter old age with a sense of delight and heightened anticipation. The commercial hard-sell of the "Golden Years" or "Golden Age" is a bit euphoric, I feel, and contains an aspect of denial of the very real adjustments needed during this particular period of life.

The aged, now considered a minority group in this culture, comprise that ever expanding group of persons aged sixty-five years or older; the majority of whom reside in the community. Although considered by the rest of the culture to be a minority group and to be set apart, the elderly do not seem to perceive themselves in that manner entirely. Puner's study (1974) confirms what many of us have frequently observed: elderly persons do not perceive themselves as "old" (p. 7). There appears to be a denial or perhaps an inability to conceptualize oneself as old. It is almost as if one has experienced one's inner self, one's feelings, one's sense of self for so long in a more or less constant manner that the external and physical aspect of oneself is assumed to have remained constant. Which is to say, ageless. Individuals often report a feeling of disbelief and amazement when they look in a mirror and see a wrinkled face staring back at them. An example of this apparent denial or unawareness of oneself as old was provided by a friend's description of her ninety-four year old mother-in-law's protestations of having to live in a nursing home "with all of those *old* people!"

INFLUENCE OF STEREOTYPES ON
HEALTH CARE

The provision of health care, and specifically nursing care, is generally influenced by the aforementioned stereotypes of the elderly that exist culturally and within the health care professions. By definition, stereotyping of the aged as a group allows for no individuality and prohibits the use of critical judgment by those who hold these fixed perceptions. In short, stereotypes prevent our seeing an elderly person as a unique human being with very individualized needs, wishes, and goals. If the caregiver holds certain stereotypes of the aged, such as "old people just wait to die," or "old people are basically dependent and helpless," then these stereotypes will carry with them a set of expectations about the patient's behavior and level of functioning. If low level expectations are held by the caregiver then these will be communicated to the aged patient, verbally or nonverbally. A patient, picking up the message that he is *not* expected to regain his ability to walk without assistance will, in all probability, lose hope that he can achieve independent mobility and give up any effort to do so. How often have we been witness to an intimate family scene where a well-meaning relative continually reinforces to an elderly member that he should just rest. "Poor dear, you're really too frail to do all this." All too soon, the elderly person who considered that he was doing just fine begins to believe that, indeed, he must be worse off than he thought!

Stereotypes beget stereotypes. The tragic outcome is that the elderly are continually reminded that they must comply with the expected social role of an aged person. They get the message that they must not deviate too far from the norm or they will be humorously chided "back into their place."

In very subtle ways the elderly are reminded of the "myths" of aging, as described by Butler (1974). Some of the primary myths of aging that Butler holds to be untrue and largely unfair are those of the overrated significance of chronological versus biological aging, lack of productivity associated with old age, inevitable disengagement or withdrawal from life, increasing rigidity with age, increased pacificity or calmness, and, finally, senility. The product and process of stereotyping the aged and the resultant discrimination is encompassed in the now widely used term "ageism" as coined by Butler in 1968 (pp. 529–35). If we are to provide adequate nursing care for our elderly patients, it is necessary for us to identify the degree of ageism that each inherited and attempt to correct, as much as possible, these stereotypes through increased knowledge, skill, experience with the aged, and increased self-understanding.

PROBLEM AREAS OF AGING

A common title for the developmental phase of old age is "senescence." Jackel (1975) discusses the three categories of problems of senescence; physical, psychological, and socioeconomic. Within each of these categories the major recurring theme is loss and the need for the senescent individual to adjust somehow to continually deteriorating abilities and decreasing opportunities (pp. 431–45).

The literature is replete with information concerning the many physical and physiological changes during the aging process, although the rate of change may vary from individual to individual. There are changes in vision due to loss of elasticity of the lens. These changes and the subsequent aids or prostheses needed for improving vision may limit social participation or cause damage to the individual's self-esteem. Visual problems and the need for appropriate prostheses may cause difficulties in any stage of life, but in the aged the result is intensified because of the cumulative nature of the losses. In youth, one loss, while still felt, can be either absorbed or compensated for by other assets. There comes a time in life, in old age, where it seems "everything goes" and there is little for which to be grateful.

Changes in auditory functioning can result in the misperception of background noises, which, in turn, may lead to an increased sense of social isolation. Total or partial loss of hearing most frequently results in an increase of suspicions about what is going on around one. It is unfortunate that this increase in suspiciousness is often attributed to either senility or mental illness when, in reality, it is often a direct result of impaired hearing. The nurse caring for elderly patients ought to be sensitive to this possibility and anticipate the patient's possible need for clarification, increased volume, or written explanations. It is very difficult to feel a part of a social group if the person cannot fully understand the communication going on around him. It is helpful if nurses anticipate this as a possible problem and can clarify the need with the patient before he becomes frustrated from asking questions or gives up and withdraws.

Other physical changes to which the elderly person may respond emotionally are decreased sensitivity to pain, decreased elasticity of the skin which promotes wrinkling, decreased physical stamina, and a decreased acuity in the sense of taste and smell. All of these physical changes elicit emotional reactions and greatly influence a person's desire and ability to interact effectively with the immediate interpersonal environment.

There is little agreement in the literature concerning the specific intellectual losses or changes in senescence. Obviously, chronic illness, organic brain impairment, or trauma could influence intellectual functioning. It has been suggested that the greatest inhibitors to intellectual functioning may be the anxiety or depression that the elderly person experiences at the time of testing.

A third category of problems occurring during the period of senescence consists of social and economic stresses. Perhaps these losses are the most visible: the loss of family, peers, lodging, social status, and meaningful activity or employment. I might add here that the loss of family or friends need not be through death. One may experience the loss of a spouse due to a physical disability in that spouse which prohibits any close communication. For example, an elderly woman may grieve for the companionship of a husband who is either deaf or has a severe memory deficit which makes verbal communication of shared feelings and concerns impossible.

As unlikely as it seems, the possible loss of a spouse through divorce was made clear in a story related to me by a psychiatrist. The psychiatrist was called for consultation at a home for the aged because an elderly woman wished to divorce her husband. The couple, both in their eighties, had been residents in this home for a few years. The wife was, of course, considered to be mentally ill or emotionally disturbed because she wanted to divorce her husband of sixty years. This couple's children were understandably upset by their mother's decision and had requested that the psychiatrist be called. When asked by the psychiatrist why, after sixty years of marriage, after bearing and raising their children, after having shared a lifetime of experiences with her husband, did she at this stage of life want to divorce him? The woman replied, "Enough is enough!"

The aged not only have to contend with specific losses, but also with the cultural attitude toward aging, which generally has been described as hostile. Gormely (1977) explains the hostile response as a defense against the fear of seeing our future selves in the aged person. In short, to see an elderly person—to experience him/her—is to grieve for our future selves. We turn away, avoid, and have contempt for what we fear will happen to us (pp. 43–124).

As discussed frequently in the literature, there is no accepted social role for the aged in this culture other than that of social isolate. Indeed, the aged have just gained legislative support to continue in the role of employee past age sixty-five if they so choose. According to Butler and Lewis (1977), higher social status and position is afforded the elderly individual who is well blessed by particular institutional or social factors. For example, the elderly person is viewed more favorably in a low productive economy that has strong religious and sacred traditions and strong familial bonds. The individual's possession of needed knowledge and skills and ownership of property also grants him higher status. This is all too evident in our culture where the worst position of all is to be old and poor and ugly (p. 23).

It is very difficult for the aged in the American culture to achieve a strong sense of social stability and esteem due to their inability to gain recognition for knowledge, skills, or any meaningful contributions. As discussed by Leaf (1973), people who no longer have a necessary role to play in the social and economic life of their society generally deteriorate rapidly. There may be too many losses too soon, with not enough support for adjustment to take place (pp. 44–52).

REACTIONS TO LOSSES

Some common emotional reactions to aging and its associated losses are discussed by Butler and Lewis (1977) and Linn (1975). Perhaps one of the most common responses is that of grief for whatever the loss has been; spouse, job, bodily function, or social status. This is similar to the grief reaction in all persons, except that for the elderly there is less of an opportunity to reinstate the lost object or to compromise and regain some of the lost gratification elsewhere. The grieving reaction generally follows a predictable pattern: initially shock, disbelief or denial; this is followed by severe emotional pain as the reality of the loss hits; then by a transient sense of unreality, possibly with delusions or a preoccupation with the lost object. There are often feelings of guilt with anger and irritability that are sometimes displaced onto friends or family members. There may be purposeless movements, sleeping and eating disturbances, and a withdrawal from social involvements.

Ordinarily a grief reaction may last a month or two before it begins to lessen. Ideally, it is resolved in six months to a year by an adaptation to the loss and reinvestment of interest and energy in the external world. Morbid or exaggerated forms of grieving may occur in which the period of grief is prolonged or even becomes chronic. This is often the case with the grief work of the elderly who are unable to replace the lost desired objects, relationships, or state of health. It must be kept in mind, however, that some losses of the elderly are not abrupt but come on gradually, such as some decrease in physical strength or function. Losses of this nature, under favorable conditions, may be adjusted to gradually or unconsciously compensated for so that the shock of the loss is never experienced by the person. On the other hand, with the aging process comes the acceleration of physical deterioration, which may be experienced as a more sudden loss. Thus it is my belief that even though there are gradually experienced losses in aging there comes a time when the realization of the cumulative effect of the losses becomes acute.

Grieving in the aged brings with it an intensification of the guilt experienced by others of younger ages. The literature on aging identifies this as being related to the normal review of one's life that is a common task during the later stage of life. Guilt may also be related to having outlived friends and colleagues, from no longer having a job or being actively involved in the work force; that is, "not carrying one's own weight."

Grief in anyone always brings with it an element of loneliness, but in the case of the elderly individual, the loneliness is often intensified by the fear that there is no one left with whom to relate. There are few outlets for many of the elderly; seldom enough to meet their emotional needs. The person experiencing a certain amount of social and emotional isolation may begin to focus inward more and more. Anxiety can intensify; especially anxiety of the free-floating nature, .as well as anxieties related to having to adjust to many drastic changes in life style and abilities. It is during this time that anxiety often arises out of identification with the recall of elderly parents. Suddenly the fears of dying in the same manner, of the same illness, at the same age, emerge. It is common to hear older individuals talking about deceased parents; comparing themselves to their parents; especially as the comparison relates to longevity.

Another form of grief that closely relates to the situation of the aged individual is that of anticipatory grief. Anticipatory grief is the process of grieving in advance of the loss. This is a type of grief not frequently identified with the aging process because so many of us are in a state of denial about our own aging process for so long. To openly admit to aging—our own ultimate aging—would be to begin to grieve in advance for losses of the anticipated future. On the one hand, the anticipatory grief process may enable us to better adjust to the losses when they do occur by having prepared us in advance for substitute gratifications. On the other hand, if we spend the present mourning the future we may lose out on the enjoyment of the present which is so indispensable for storing up fulfilling memories.

Loneliness, another possible reaction to aging, represents one of the most uncomfortable emotions to be endured. Weiss (1973) differentiates depression from loneliness and discusses the loneliness resulting from emotional as well as social isolation. He makes the distinction between depression and loneliness in terms of dealing with the lost object. In loneliness, according to Weiss, there is an urge to correct the feeling of something being missing by moving toward another need-fulfilling relationship. In depression, on the other hand, one gives in to the feeling of missing the lost one. Grief is viewed as the *experience* of the loss of a cherished object rather than a *reaction* to the absence of a valued person or object.

Weiss then differentiates between the experiences of emotional social isolation. He stresses the point that in the experience of emotional isolation there is no close emotional involvement. It cannot be eliminated except through the development of a close emotional relationship or by the return of the lost one. Emotional isolation is likened to feelings of abandonment.

Social isolation, on the other hand, is viewed as a reaction to the loss of an active social matrix of objects. It is experienced as boredom, feelings of exclusion, and of not being a part of a larger group. Weiss thinks that the aged may well suffer from extreme loneliness due to a loss of specific object attachments and an isolation from society's social matrix (pp. 15-22)

Townsend (1973) explores the isolation and loneliness of the aged as it relates to their degree of social contact. He finds that the aged are very susceptible to the experience of loneliness, and that while there does not appear to be a single causative factor for the loneliness, those who are more elderly, single or childless, and infirm, appear to be in the highest risk group. Other significant factors contributing to loneliness are recent (within the past five years) loss of a loved one, a change in social status or in housing, or additional circumstances such as retirement or bereavement. It is stressed that resolution of the loneliness due to social or emotional isolation is not a simple matter. It may be that the individuals involved may have to struggle to develop alternative methods of living with loneliness rather than eliminate it (pp. 175-88).

Depression, as a response to aging, is perhaps the most frequently seen reaction to the guilt, anger, and the losses of the aging process. Rubin (1975) stresses the role of self-hate in the depressions of the aged. This feeling of disgust for oneself, one's body, is especially destructive because the march of time and its resultant toll on the human body and function cannot be changed. This cycle of disgust, self-hate, and helplessness becomes entrenched and intensifies unless the individual gains help in coming to terms with himself and his life. Again, it must be kept in mind that not all individuals experience this self-hate. Those who have a healthy regard for themselves and enjoy life may never experience this painful reaction to the aging process. Rubin pleads for compassion for oneself and emphasizes the need to live within the realistic limits of one's abilities (pp. 236–37). This implies the ability to modify one's goals and expectations and to receive satisfaction in what is possible rather than in what might have been. Unfortunately, this is much easier prescribed than implemented. How does one easily relinquish goals and expectations?

FACTORS PROMOTING ADAPTATION TO AGING

The literature is replete with articles identifying those factors that promote a positive adaptation to the aging process. It has been widely accepted that such things as maintaining a useful and satisfying role or position in society, the maintenance of good physical condition, and a healthy, optimistic view of life promote a successful adaptation to aging. The problem is how to help those not so blessed to achieve some sense of fulfillment in their later years and to minimize the untoward reactions to the inevitable losses.

According to Levin (1963), loss signifies a deficiency in those external environmental or interpersonal supplies needed to provide satisfaction of drives and needs. In discussing external factors related to depression he adds that, in addition to loss, environmentally imposed physical or psychological pain, such as neglect, physical injury, ridicule, or humiliation, may influence depression. The elderly, of course, are very vulnerable to the social and cultural slights intentionally given them. To see oneself mirrored in the eyes and faces of others as hopeless, worthless, ugly and old must be painful indeed (pp. 302-7).

A third force that may underlie the depression found in some aged is that of the many restrictions and constrictions placed upon need gratification or upon those activities necessary for need gratification. Any restriction of physical activity could, therefore, contribute to depression if the restriction prevents the individual from obtaining gratifications in life. Witness the many and often subtle constraints upon the sexual activity of the elderly—especially in hospitals and nursing homes.

Although not mentioned by Levin, psychological restraint in the form of limitations placed on decision making could contribute to depression if the need for mastery or a sense of some control over one's environment is lost or interfered with. Colligan (1975) and Seligman (1975) have both stressed the theory that loss of control over one's life can lead to the loss of motivation to continue one's life. In a very real sense, the aged can die from a sense of helplessness or from a sense of loss of control over their lives.

The fourth external factor influencing depression, according to Levin (1963) is the threat of any future loss, injury, or impediment. While true for any age group, the elderly are perhaps a bit more vulnerable because the losses seem to accelerate, while the opportunities for gratification decrease and the anticipated future shortens (pp. 302-7).

Some of the events that may be most threatening to the aged are those which imply, explicitly or implicitly, abandonment by significant others, disability, suffering or pain, and death. While threatening to anyone, these events are especially destructive to the aged because there is so little time and opportunity for restitution. The elderly may more readily "give up hope" for any change unless someone is available to them for support. Unfortunately, many supportive services, including psychotherapy, are not readily available to the elderly because of the biased attitude that there is no payoff or that the aged cannot change. It has been hypothesized that the elderly, or anyone, can intuitively pick up these feelings of hopelessness and withdrawal from others. This, then, undermines their will and their hope for some relief.

It is possible for an individual to be unaware of his attachment to persons, situations, or objects and, therefore, to be unaware of the source of his depressive response regarding the lost objects. In addition to the more obvious losses one can experience, Levin (1965) proposes that there are events that can be presumed to be "loss equivalents." One such instance may be when someone else's gain or achievement is felt as envy or jealousy—as though it implied a loss to oneself. Any type of disappointment may be thought of as a loss equivalent; as something which although anticipated as gratifying, was not forthcoming. One may, therefore, feel one's wish or hope to be lost. This may result in an increased sense of oneself being diminished. It is very important, therefore, to consider both actual and perceived losses (and their anniversaries) as well as the loss equivalents in attempting to determine possible causes for depression in the aged (pp. 203-25).

PERSONALITY STYLES AND
COPING PATTERNS

Before moving to the area of planning health care for the elderly person, it may be helpful to consider what personality styles and ways of coping people may bring to the aging process. If we are able to have some framework for understanding the variables influencing styles of adaptation to aging then we may be better able to provide the needed support for the elderly individual attempting to meet his unique needs.

Neugarten, Havinghurst and Tobin (1968), discussing a study designed to describe patterns of aging, have examined three categories of data: (1) personality type, (2) the degree of social role involvement, and (3) the degree of life satisfaction. They have identified four major personality patterns, each with subgroups according to the extent of role activity and amount of life satisfaction. In other words, these authors have identified eight personality patterns of aging.

The Healthy Personality. This personality type is seen as being essentially healthy; having characteristics of openness, flexibility, and great satisfaction with their lives. Within this major group of essentially intact and integrated individuals are two subgroups. One subgroup, high in activity, tends to be able to substitute new activities for old or to be able to reorganize their patterns of activity relatively easily. The second subgroup differs only in that their activity pattern is less active and they tend to gain life satisfaction from only one or two role areas. They also substitute activities, but in a much more selective manner.

The Disengaged Personality. A second major pattern identified by Neugarten et al. is called "disengaged." These individuals are highly integrated or healthy personality types with a high degree of satisfaction in life but with a low degree of activity. This approach to aging has been called elsewhere "the rocking chair approach" to old age. These are self-directed persons who do not prefer a large social matrix within which to function. They are quite self-contained.

The Highly Defended Personality. A third major pattern described by Neugarten et al. is a highly defended approach to aging. The individuals in this group are highly achievement oriented with a great many defenses against anxiety and a great need for tight controls over their impulses. Within this major pattern, two subgroups emerge: the "holding on" and "constricted" patterns of aging. Individuals classified in the "holding on" group find aging a great threat and attempt to prolong middle age as long as possible. They are successful in maintaining a high degree of life satisfaction as long as they maintain a fairly high degree of activity. The "constricted" group represents those individuals who tend to be excessively preoccupied with the losses of the aging process and defend themselves by restricting, or narrowing, their social experiences. Their activity level is low but they can experience a high level of gratification with their lives as long as the restricted activity works to prevent them from experiencing losses.

The Passive-dependent Personality. The fourth pattern identified is that of the most passive-dependent type of individual. This pattern has two subgroups of personality types: those who seek a great deal of attention and nurturing from others to meet their very high dependency needs, and those who are apathetic. Individuals who have high dependency needs and seek a great deal of caring from others may experience an average degree of satisfaction from their lives as long as they have at least one or two other people to whom to turn for their emotional needs. Those individuals whose personalities and approaches to life would be termed "apathetic" are generally quite passive people. They have a low activity pattern and generally are not very satisfied with their lives. It is as though they wait for others to provide them with satisfactions rather than to exert any energy to help to provide their own satisfactions from life.

The Disorganized Personality. The final group is described as "disorganized." Members of this group evidence a great deal of impairment of physical and psychological functioning. They are, however, able to maintain themselves in the com-

munity but evidence a minimum amount of social involvement and experience little satisfaction.

Neugarten et al. conclude that the pattern of aging that a
person demonstrates is essentially the same pattern of living
that he has followed throughout his life. The essential point
is that individuals adapt to life in a fairly consistent pattern
according to their many unique needs (pp. 173-77). This is
not to imply, however, that if an individual has a low life
satisfaction, that there is little that can be done to alter the
aged person's sense of loneliness, grief, and depression. There
is a current emphasis in the popular and professional literature upon increased knowledge and skill needed to help
remove the elderly from the abyss of social isolation to which
they have been relegated. Kaplan (1976) emphasizes the
social and cultural aspects of aging and stresses the need for
change in the cultural meaning of aging and the aged. Any
less ambitious a focus would promote smaller, shorter-term
changes on the social level—on the level of our everyday
personal exchanges and relationships (p. 346).

NURSING CARE CONSIDERATIONS

Currently the literature reflects professional concern related to the care of the elderly. The public literature abounds
with discussions of the many injustices to the aged and with
pleas for increased social awareness to the plight of the aged
in this culture. Maggie Kuhn, who, at age 72, started the
protest group called the Gray Panthers is currently bringing
to public and legal view the many subtle ways that derogatory
attitudes about the elderly are being reinforced.

Self-help books directed toward those currently called
aged and those who will someday become aged have been
written by such current authors as Comfort (1976) and
Galton (1975). Comfort focuses upon providing certain
strategies to deal with a culture not yet accepting of the aged,

while Galton proposes a "how to" approach to the restoration of some measure of physical and mental functioning to the lives of the aged in such a way as to stir enthusiasm and hope in the reader. An exceptionally fine example from the current literature that combines professional scope of content with a sensitivity to the needs of the family of the aged individual is the work by Silverstone and Hyman (1976). The proliferation of books on how to age successfully or how to help someone else live effectively with the aging process indicates that there is a great concern in this area. Like it or not, nurses will have to give some thought to the issues involved in helping people to live with the inevitable losses, necessary adjustments, and frequent grief of growing old. This is difficult, because as one elderly patient once informed me, "You just don't think about it 'til it happens because you've never been old before."

I do believe she was right in the sense that we really *do not* know what the experience of aging is until we are aged. But this does not mean that we cannot develop some cognitive appreciation for the process from those who have studied it and from those who are living it. As in other areas of nursing, when all else fails, listen to the patient. It just may give us some clues as to what is really going on.

Help Needed by the Aged to Adjust to Loss. Perhaps the first consideration that nurses need to give to the problem of how to help the aged person adjust to grief associated with loss is to recognize that not all of them need this help. To be sure, there comes a time when physical deterioration is so great that one needs to be taken care of by others. However, it is important to recognize that not every elderly person necessarily grieves for the many losses previously discussed. As one older colleague shared with me, "Your expectations and values and priorities change as you grow older, so of course you don't miss those things. I can't honestly say that I 'grieve' for the fact that I can no longer climb that pine tree out there." If one can adjust to losses gradually, one does not mourn their absence. What she did not add was that it is often we who project our anticipated grief onto the elderly person. This colleague, along with Maggie Kuhn, illustrates the "integrated" style of aging discussed earlier in this chapter. In all probability, although this type of individual will inevitably experience loss and will grieve, the grief will be of the relatively uncomplicated type and will run its course in six months to a year if there is some support from others. The one major problem may be the loss of a long-time spouse. Current studies indicate this stress may negatively influence the individual's health, and the period of grieving may take approximately two years rather than the usually stipulated twelve months (Parks, 1972, pp. 176–77).

It is important, then, for the nurse to assess the individual's previous pattern of adaptation. Was it well integrated, was it the rocking chair approach to life, the highly threatened and defended pattern, the passive-dependent approach, or the disorganized pattern of adjustment? This knowledge will enable the nurse to predict which individual might have a complicated or protracted grieving reaction to aging. It would appear evident that those persons who have fewer resources with which to deal with loss, that is, poor physical health, low life satisfaction, few object relationships coupled with a need for them, and poor material resources, would be at high risk. Individuals with low activity, low life satisfaction, and little hope are likely to be in most need of intervention. If the grieving process is protracted it may become chronic or lead to suicide in the elderly—a relatively common phenomenon.

It is important to assess the patient's perceptions and feelings about himself and the aging phenomenon. Frank signs of depression are easy to identify by their mood components and physiological manifestations. Irritability, confusion, apathy, hypochrondriasis, or hyperactivity may be indications of a masked depression that requires further validation.

Of particular significance in assessment of the elderly is any history of losses: homes, family members, surgeries, or loss of some aspect of bodily function. Losses of this type, especially if they have occurred within the past two years, may result in depression. Grieving over a loss is usually resolved within two years. If not, it becomes chronic and may be expressed through any of the depressive responses.

Depression in the elderly is generally related to losses, unresolved grief, or to possible metabolic changes in old age. Supportive counseling, the use of antidepressant medication, or psychotherapy can be helpful if the depression is severe or if the elderly person has verbalized or attempted suicide. It is needless for the elderly to have to endure the pain of depression just because some health professionals feel it is a waste of time to treat the elderly. The elderly *can* respond to treatment, but only if the treatment is offered.

The depressive response to aging is one commonly seen in any type of care setting. Should the patient be suicidal, it is obviously important to monitor his behavior closely and help him to verbally share his feelings. Assessment here should also include a history of losses, interpersonal and social resources, previous suicide attempts, and previous coping patterns. If the patient is placed on any of the tricyclic medications (such as Elavil, Tofranil, or Sinequan) they cannot expect any clinical results for three weeks and ought to be monitored closely for the many possible side effects of these drugs. Some common side effects of the tricyclics are hypotension, or hypertension, mania or hyperactivity, extrapyramidal symptoms (e.g., hand tremors, muscle rigidity, stiff neck) or confusion, to name a few.

Burnside (1969) stresses the need to get patients to verbally share their feelings, fears, and anger to begin to resolve these. An important point is also made that often the patient does not connect the feelings he is experiencing with the actual loss. He may need to be told that he is depressed or grieving, if indeed he is, and told that he *has* suffered losses sufficient to warrant those feelings. Oftentimes just having a word symbol or name to attach to a feeling and some glimmer of cognitive understanding will promote an initial sense of control or mastery. This, in turn, eliminates some of the fear and anxiety that the person is experiencing (pp. 416–27).

Awareness of One's Own Feelings. To understand the needs and emotional reactions of the aging individual to losses, the nurse must first be open to experiencing her own fears and feelings about aging and the aged. If we are not open to our feelings of fear, distrust, contempt, or pity, then we will be unable to adequately emphathize with either the aging person or with his family and acquaintances who need and deserve our care. Kastenbaum (1971) has devised a way, through artificial situations, to help young persons prepare for aging by helping them experience some of the losses and frustrations of old age. I am not certain that I would advocate this sort of preparation for getting in touch with one's feelings about old age. There are other ways that we can increase our self-awareness in this area: through concentrated introspection, structured group sessions, or continued educational opportunities, for example. The point is, we need, as honestly as possible, to come to grips with our individual feelings and cultural stereotypes regarding the aged; our nursing care of the elderly patient should not be inhibited by any predispositions. Harrison (1971) succinctly states that the central issue in the art of nursing practice involves separation of our projections about the elderly patient from our performance. Nursing care should be based instead upon the individual patient's own perceptions and style of life (p. 46). A creative idea, if only nursing can begin to implement it!

It is all too evident that geriatrics is not a popular field in medicine, psychiatry, or nursing. In protest of the deplorable neglect of the medical and emotional problems of the aged, Galton (1975) has written about the "clinical caretakers" of

medicine who have been guilty of seeing the elderly as untreatable and neglecting their emotional reactions to long-
term illness. These "clinical caretakers" seem to tolerate
caring for the elderly only because they can greedily collect
the Medicaide and Medicare payments. Galton indicated that
a report of an American Medical Association committee on
aging gave a name to the type of medical practice that bars
treatment to the aged. It is called "condescension medicine"
(p. 11). Elderly patients either do not get accepted for
treatment—a very real current problem, by the way—or the
elderly are accepted but given only superficial bandaid treatment, a pat on the head, and a knowing wink at the relative,
which is supposed to convey the shared and condescending
truth that, "Of course we both know it is all in her head—
old folks complain a lot." Recently, in seeking a medical
referral for an aged relative, I learned that the first question
to ask was, "Do you treat elderly people?" After six months
of searching for competent, concerned medical care for my
relative, I learned that what might have been a treatable
carcinoma was finally diagnosed as untreatable.

Physicians are not the only health professionals to practice condescension. Sometimes nurses are caught up in the
same stereotypic attitudes of futility, hopelessness, and
contempt toward that which they fear. It is not only the
elderly who must learn to modify values and standards.
Perhaps nurses, too, need to assess their own feelings, attitudes, stereotypes.

Competencies Needed for Work with the Elderly. Moos
(1977) identified four areas of competence needed for staff
dealing with persons with any chronic condition. I believe his
study is directly applicable to the staff dealing with aged
individuals. One of these areas of competence has been discussed: that of awareness of the previous coping patterns
used by the elderly patient so that we can work to reinforce

these patterns if they are adaptive in the current situation. A second area of competence identified by Moos is a real understanding of and appreciation for the time it takes to work through the resolution of a loss (p. 18). As I mentioned earlier, reports of recent research on the grief and mourning process, especially as it relates to the loss of a spouse, indicate that it may take two years to effectively resolve this grief. This is much longer than we previously anticipated. At any rate, if we are impatient, or cut off the feelings related to the grieving process, the patient may never be able to fully resolve his loss.

The third area of competence identified by Moos is an understanding of what environmental supports, or lack of them, might facilitate or hinder adaptation. It is necessary to know what support systems, human or nonhuman, may exist for each patient and how we can incorporate them into our care. And, finally, Moos reiterates what so many other authors have stressed, that it is mandatory that the care giver have an understanding of his or her own feelings and reactions to the aged and infirm (pp. 17-20).

When we emphasize that nurses must understand the previous coping patterns of elderly patients, what exactly should the nurse look for? Moos indicates that all people facing a life crisis strive to maintain emotional equilibrium, to go through the crisis with as much positive esteem and sense of mastery and control as possible. They want to maintain relationships with significant others, to mourn their losses, and to prepare themselves for an uncertain future. One could look at these as tasks to be accomplished in going through a "chronic crisis." The nurse could use her awareness of these adaptive tasks as a guideline for general areas of needed support with aged individuals who evidence difficulty in emotional stability, are depressed, have a negative feeling about themselves, feel everything is out of their control, or have a breakdown in social relationships (pp. 9-10).

Dealing with Chronic Grief. Moos addresses the many ways that individuals attempt to deal with chronic grief; ways that may be more or less constructive. Some individuals, in an attempt to maintain a sense of control, deny or minimize the impact of their loss by somatizing, displacing or projecting their fears or anger. A seemingly healthier approach is to use intellectual resources to handle stress. The person may want to ask questions or read to gain additional information. As mentioned earlier, cognitive awareness and understanding often increases one's sense of mastery and control, which in turn decreases one's sense of helplessness.

Information sharing as an intervention can give a great sense of mastery to the elderly person who is so often robbed of control of his right to make or participate in making his own decisions. Unfortunately, the elderly often are not even informed of major developments or changes affecting their lives. A painful example of this occurred when I had to tell a hospitalized elderly man recovering from abdominal surgery that no one in his family wanted to care for him and that he had no where to go upon discharge. His family had moved his belongings out of his rented flat, had rerented the flat, and had stored his belongings while he was in the hospital having surgery. What an unbearable assault upon one's self-esteem and feelings of competence! While the situation did not turn out well, at least he was able to gather the information he needed to begin to deal with the situation. I experienced great pain in answering, directly and honestly, his many questions.

Other individuals, according to Moos, reach out for support and reassurance. People who tend to be action oriented do well if they can master or learn new procedures or techniques, such as diet or motor control. The nurse can assist patients in setting small, attainable goals which give them a sense of achievement and, therefore, mastery and competence. There is also a psychological variation of this in the area of helping the patient to learn to anticipate alternatives and outcomes painful experiences I have had. It would have been infinitely easier to have dissuaded him from this pilgrimage or to have refused to drive him. But some grief must be experienced, shared, and borne. One must be open to that, too, if one is to be open to life.

We must not stifle the grieving of our patients. How they manage it is ultimately dependent upon what resources they have and upon what adaptive patterns they bring into the situation. We cannot prevent them from entering the process of grief in order to protect ourselves against the pain. So too with depression. The nurse might focus with the elderly on esteem-building activities: the restoration of some sense of mastery or control over their lives, the restoration of significant memorabilia or objects, or simply human contact—lending an ear to their feelings. In order for individuals to "come up" from depression they need someone to be there—to supportively allow them to experience and express their feelings. It is esteem building to know that another person cares enough about you to be with you during painful periods. These activities can serve to elevate self-esteem and where there is a high level of self-esteem there is little depression.

Supporting the Aged Person's Need for Mastery/Control. A sense of mastery or competence is significant to one's effective adaptation to the long-term crisis of aging. A sense of control or mastery over even a portion of one's life is a strengthening feeling, and, as such diminishes that most destructive of feelings, namely, helplessness. Loss of a sense of control or mastery over one's body or bodily functions can be one of the most degrading experiences for a person. Old age, illness, and disability rob us of a sense of control over our destiny. Indeed, nursing care often removes the element of control in decision making from the patient. The elderly have so many losses that they need to feel mastery over some part of their situation, if only on an intellectual level.

of certain choices. An important aim for pe
chronic stress is to find some pattern or m
existence. Anticipatory mourning may be
that is, the beginning of the grief work pr
loss. Often this is a difficult theme for nurses
it triggers their own fears of loss. But, it is
that the patient be allowed this expression.

A helpful framework for the nurse to u
previous personality and adaptive patterns t
used and thus avoid jumping to conclusio
long-enduring adjustment patterns just beca
measure up to the nurse's expectations. Th
intervention is on those aspects of disturbe
evidence an unintegrated personality, a
aspects of the environment which do not
functioning and life satisfaction.

The main thing I would like to stress a
grieving in the elderly is *not* to stifle it. As
be for nurses and family members, elde
support in experiencing and expressing gri
in escaping from it. An elderly man in a nu
his family's aid in getting out. In truth, he
to be there since he was self-sufficient and
tress, but none of his immediate family
children had offered him a home but this
from his long-time residential area. One
stepchildren to drive him to visit a numbe
neighbors. One-by-one he asked each of
take him in as a boarder or rent him a sm
one they apologetically came up with re
rationalizations why they could not do
despair he felt was mirrored in his eyes, k
sense of dignity since he knew he had a
final attempt to gain acceptance and co
he had to do even though it resulted in
and allow him to do this was one of th

There are some specific areas that nurses need to consider in becoming sensitive to the needs of elderly patients. We can help them regain a sense of mastery of body function, for example, through appropriate exercises. Or the extremely confused patient may be helped immeasurably through a decrease in external stimuli and consistency in nurses assigned to his care, in order to help him regain a sense of mastery over his environment, no matter how limited. We can examine how much mastery we unnecessarily deprive patients of by identifying how we exclude them from decision making about their care. We can also identify and alter ways we deprive them of productive activity or even of their possessions. Part of the elderly person's preoccupation with money has to do with his fears of losing mastery or independence in a highly materialistic society. If one loses control over one's money, then one has, in a sense, lost all mastery over one's fate.

Life Review.   One process that occurs periodically throughout life, but more often in old age, and can have esteem-building potential is the review of one's life. The life review is a naturally occurring return to conscious awareness of past experiences, regrets, wishes, and unresolved conflicts (Butler, 1968). Ideally, once reviewed, feelings about these experiences can be resolved and reintegrated into the personality (pp. 486–89). The danger is that reviewed material may increase guilt, depression, and negative feelings. Or, this spontaneously occurring phenomenon may have adaptive and constructive potential in that it can provide increased understanding of the person's existence, the emergence of new, adaptive feelings, as well as a source of gratification based upon past experiences. The process of reminiscing can often bring about the life review. Reminiscing has been widely written about as a therapeutic intervention in and of itself. It can sometimes be difficult for the nurse or younger person to listen to, however. We tend to be future oriented and become impatient when the elderly patient wishes to focus on the past.

Ebersole (1976) has written about therapeutic group techniques utilizing the reminiscences of the aged. Her rationale is that reminiscing not only increases the self-esteem of the participants, but also increases social interaction, increases a sense of belonging as a means of combating the isolation of the aged, and enhances the participant's interpersonal awareness (pp. 214–30). Reminiscing is an important aspect of putting one's life in order. An example of a form of reminiscing is seen in the written memoirs of the famous. These memoirs are written more for the author than for the audience. In the case of elderly patients, this activity should be encouraged.

The nurse must identify the degree of independence in activities of daily living and the range of functioning possible for the elderly person. It is also important to assess the degree of alertness and coordination so as to provide for consistency in care. If a patient is mildly confused the nurse might find alternatives to hot tub baths since hot water dilates peripheral blood vessels and decreases the blood supply to the brain, causing further dizziness and confusion.

Of great importance in assessment is the individual's motivation to maintain or regain independent functioning. An awareness of elderly patients' levels of functioning in these areas will help us to plan intervention and care that will not rob individuals of their much needed self-reliance and inner sustainment which is necessary for a heightened sense of self-esteem.

Review of Financial Resources. The last area of assessment must, of necessity, include the financial resources of the elderly individual. This to a great degree determines the kind of care available to him or her.

Goals of Intervention. What then are general goals of psychologic intervention for the aged individual? We have discussed the prime areas of concern: depression, loss and grief, and loneliness. Goldfarb (1974) indicates that treatment, care, and prevention can be approached both early and late in the aging process by focusing on replacements, substitutions, or compromises to replace what was lost, by guarding against loss of a sense of mastery, by dealing with feelings of helplessness, and by dealing with the painful feelings as these develop (p. 839). The appropriate use of support and reassurance can help the patient feel less abandoned and helpless. The elderly patient can benefit from the interpersonal relationship with the helping person. He makes of the relationship what he most needs at that time—support, validation, or a sense of worthwhileness. Graded tasks or behavioral assignments can be given to further provide the patient with a sense of mastery.

Battin, Arkin, Gerber, and Wiener (1975) focus on a treatment plan designed to deal solely with grief and bereavement in the aged. Their intervention, which is psychiatrically based, lasted six months and focused on a series of therapeutic progressions aimed at encouraging expression of feelings of pain, anger, and the finality of the lost object. The aim was to help the elderly person deal with how he would retain the lost object and still deal effectively with the realities of everyday life. This approach can be implemented as long as the patient determines the pace and is permitted to lead, at his own rate, into areas of painful feelings (pp. 292–302). It must be remembered that not all individuals can, or should, resolve the grief for a lost person, or situation, or body function. Steger (1976) discusses the value of the "sick role" in avoiding painful feelings of loneliness and in giving a social "niche." For some elderly, then, this may be their only viable alternative (p. 71).

What we, as nurses, can do is to attempt to combat those debilitating external forces of loss, insecurity, and restraint on the elderly, and focus, above all, on doing all we can to help them maintain some sense of control and mastery, if only through the intellectual processes which govern their lives and situations. Until such a time as cultural values and norms change in such a way as to grant a degree of respectability to the aged, we can at least work to help them to accept their necessary dependence upon us with a measure of grace and dignity.

REFERENCES

Battin, D.; Arkin, A.; Gerber, I.; and Wiener, A. 1975. Coping and vulnerability among the aged bereaved. In *Bereavement: its psychosocial aspects,* eds. B. Schoenberg, I. Gerber, A. Wiener, A. H. Kutscher, D. Peretz, and A. C. Carr. New York: Columbia University Press.

Burnside, I. M. 1969. Griefwork in the aged patient. *Nursing Forum* 8:416-27.

Butler, R. 1968. The life review: an interpretation of reminiscence in the aged. In *Middle life and aging,* ed. B. L. Neugarten. Chicago: University of Chicago Press.

——. 1974. Successful aging and the role of the life review. *Journal of the American Geriatric Society* 22:529-35.

Butler, R., and Lewis, M. I. 1977. *Aging and mental health: positive psychosocial approaches.* 2nd ed. Saint Louis: C. V. Mosby Company.

Colligan, D. 1975. That helpless feeling: the dangers of stress. *New York Magazine,* July, 28-32.

Comfort, A. 1976. *A good age.* New York: Crown Publishers, Inc.

Curtain, S. 1972. *Nobody ever died of old age: in praise of old people—in outrage of their loneliness.* Boston: Little, Brown and Company, An Atlantic Monthly Press Book.

Ebersole, P. P. 1976. Reminiscing and group psychotherapy with the aged. In *Nursing and the aged,* ed. I. M. Burnside. New York: McGraw-Hill.

Galton, L. 1975. *Don't give up on your aging parent.* New York: Crown Publishers, Inc.

Goldfarb, A. I. 1975. Depression in the old and aged. In *The nature and treatment of depression*, eds. F. F. Flach and S. C. Draghi. New York: Wiley and Sons.

——. 1974. Minor maladjustments of the aged. In *The American handbook of psychiatry*, volume 3, 2nd ed. eds. S. Arieti, and E. Brody. New York: Basic Books, Inc.

Gormely, S. 1977. Love among the aged. *Toronto Life*, March, 43–124.

Harrison, C. 1971. The patient that is and is not. *Journal of Nursing Administration* 1:46.

Jackel, M. M. 1975. Senescence. In *Personality development and deviation*, ed. G. H. Wiedman. New York: International Universities Press.

Kahn, R. L.; Zarit, S. H.; Hilbert, N. M.; and Niedereke, G. 1975. Memory complaint and impairment in the aged: the effect of depression and arterial brain function. *Archives of General Psychiatry* 32:1569–73.

Kaplan, D. M. 1976. Freud and the coming of age. *Bulletin of the Menninger Clinic* 40:346.

Kastenbaum, R. 1971. Getting there ahead of time. *Psychology Today* 5:52–84.

Leaf, A. 1973. Getting old. *Scientific America* 229:44–52.

Levin, S. 1965. Depression in the aged. In *Geriatric psychiatry*, eds. M. A. Berezin and S. H. Cath. New York: International Universities Press.

——. 1963. Depression in the aged: a study of the salient external factors. *Geriatrics* 18:302–7.

Linn, L. 1975. Neurologic aspects of aging. In *Personality development and deviation*, ed. G. H. Wiedman. New York: International Universities Press.

Moos, R. H., 1977. *Coping with physical illness*. New York: Plenum Medical Book Company.

Neugarten, G. L.; Havinghurst, R. J.; and Tobin, S. S. 1968. Personality patterns in aging. In *Middle life and aging*, ed. B. L. Neugarten. Chicago: University of Chicago Press.

Palmore, E. B. 1973. Social factors in mental illness of the aged. In *Mental illness in later life,* eds. E. W. Busse, and E. Pfieffer. Washington, D.C.: American Psychiatric Association.

Parks, C. M. 1972. *Bereavement: studies in grief in adult life.* New York: International Universities Press, Inc.

Puner, M. 1974. *To the good life: what we know about growing old.* New York: Universal Books.

Rubin, T. I. 1975. *Compassion and self-hate: an alternative to despair.* New York: Ballentine Books.

Seligman, M. E. P. 1975. *Helplessness: on depression, development and death.* San Francisco: W. H. Freeman and Company.

Silverstone, B., and Hyman, H. K. 1976. *You and your aging parent: the modern family's guide to emotional, physical and financial problems.* New York: Pantheon Books.

Steger, H. G. 1976. Understanding the psychologic factors in rehabilitation. *Geriatrics* 31:71.

Townsend, P. 1973. Isolation and loneliness in the aged. In *Loneliness: the experience of emotional and social isolation,* ed. R. S. Weiss. Cambridge, Massachusetts: M.I.T. Press.

Weiss, R. S. 1973. *Loneliness: the experience of emotional and social isolation.* Cambridge, Massachusetts: M.I.T. Press.

PART THREE

Part Three includes two chapters which at first glance may seem unrelated to the nursing care of individuals who are grieving the loss of physical health and/or function. However, if one views hope as the opposite of grief, then it becomes exceedingly important for nurses to understand how hope can be fostered in the grieving person whether that person be patient, family member, or caregiver. Likewise, the nurse who works with the long-term patient who is grieving his losses needs to be aware of strategies for personal support. This is essential if the nurse is to maintain her satisfaction with nursing.

Chapter 7, "Nursing and the Concept of Hope," examines the components of hope and attempts to translate these into a "language" for nursing practice. The need for nurses to be risk takers as well as responsible, accountable professional care providers is stressed.

Chapter 8, "The Burnout Syndrome in Nurses," considers the humanness of nurses as individuals who react to stress. Nowhere in nursing is there a greater need to understand the circumstances that produce stress in nurses than among those nurses who work with patients with long-term illness or disabilities—and especially those patients who are in the throes of grief associated with their losses. Too often texts

address only what nurses should do for others.
The emotionally depleted nurse is of questionable value in patient care. This chapter takes a
close look at options that, if taken, can avoid
such depletion.

CHAPTER SEVEN

Nursing and the Concept of Hope

Jean A. Werner-Beland

INTRODUCTION

Gabriel Marcel's essay, "Sketch of a Phenomonology and a Metaphysic of Hope" (1962) has numerous implications for nursing practice; more specifically for nursing practice as it relates to the chronically ill and disabled who oftentimes abandon hope for despair and enter into protracted periods of grieving. This chapter is an attempt at weaving Marcel's philosophical work into an operational frame for nursing practice; especially as nursing practice relates to patients who are grieving the loss of their own health and functioning.

WISH VS. BELIEF IN HOPE

Marcel indicates that there are two elements in the concept of "I hope." First, there is a wish. Second, this wish is also accompanied by a certain belief (p. 29). This seems simple enough at first glance, and yet, a nursing assessment that

169

takes into account only the wish and fails to explore with the patient the nature of the belief held in relation to that wish, is apt to misperceive and underestimate the complexity of the problem. In work with patients we are often confronted with seemingly incomprehensible situations. We teach a patient what we think he needs to know in order to sustain or regain health, the patient gives every indication of under-standing what he has been told and then behaves in a manner contrary to prescribed health-sustaining measures. Why? One reason being proposed here is that the wish and the belief are not in correspondence with each other, and this discrepancy has not been recognized by the health care providers.

For example, in Chapter 4 Delaney-Naumoff cites the case of a man who, after suffering a severe myocardial infarct, went against the advice given by the health care providers and, subsequently, died in the cab of his truck. This case illustrates the wish-belief discrepancy. The man wished he were well and able to work and support his family. His belief was that he would only be a burden on his family. He believed his family would be better off without him because if he were dead they would have his insurance and greater financial security. The end result was that he behaved in a manner that corresponded with the fulfillment of his belief.

In such situations hindsight may teach us something about future interventions. What might have happened if the family had been able to convince the man in our example that he was of more worth to them than a big house in a wealthy sub-urb? What if they had recognized his belief and had been able to effectively communicate that they were willing to make a few material sacrifices in order to have him around? That is, what if it had been possible to bring his belief more in line with understanding how he might eventually attain his wish? Maybe things would have ended differently. All of this specu-lation would, of course, depend upon the patient's willing-ness and ability to change his belief in the face of other evidence.

The important point is that other evidence needs to be made available to the patient or he is apt to remain locked into a self-destructive belief. Nursing needs to assume responsibility for exploring ways of bringing this evidence to the patient's awareness. However, increasing the patient's awareness can only be accomplished when attention is paid to the belief component as well as the wish component. Even then, as with the man in the truck, there may be results contrary to our desires, but not because we failed to include an important component of care. We simply do not control everyone's fate.

Marcel also apeaks of the concept "I hope" in time of trial as being directed toward deliverance from the captivity imposed by that trial. Such trials we are told:

> invariably imply the impossibility, not necessarily of moving or even acting in a manner which is relatively free, but *of rising to a certain fullness of life, which may be in the realms of sensation or even thought in a strict sense of the word* (p. 30).

To be removed from one's normal life style or sphere of activities because of illness or disability is, in a sense, a captivity that carries with it all the ingredients for further alienation. Marcel states:

> This is illustrated in the case of the invalid for whom the word health arouses a wealth of associations generally unsuspected by those who are well. Yet, at the same time, we must determine not only what is positive but what is illusory in this idea of health which the sick man cherishes (p. 31).

As with the wish-belief discrepancy, the further apart are the facts and illusions related to an individual's concept of health, the more he becomes a captive of his situation; and the more likely he is to remain in anguish because of it.

Therefore, when we speak of acceptance in nursing, we are really addressing the reduction of the psychological "space" between the wishes and beliefs (or the facts and illusions) that a person holds relative to his health.

As Zuzich (Chapter 5) points out, the parent who is unable to resolve the conflict between a fantasied "perfect" baby and the reality of a retarded child cannot learn to accept the real child as a human being who has assets as well as limitations. The same notion holds true for the individual who becomes ill or disabled. If he or she cannot resolve the distance between what is a fantasied image of self (as based upon an image of self as what once was, as well as values related to perfection) and what now is, then efforts to assist this person to accept his limitations and to discover previously untapped personal resources will not occur. It becomes a vital bit of data in nursing assessment and in the understanding of patients' reponses to recognize that on the one hand the patient is wishing he were perfect and that everything that was previously possible for him would be still possible, while on the other hand clinging to the belief that nothing is possible. Work on grief resolution will be unsuccessful as long as this wish-belief conflict remains.

Helping patients resolve the wish-belief dilemma becomes a tricky problem for nursing intervention. While we do not think it constructive for a patient to cling to unrealistic fantasies or wishes, neither do we view beating the person over the head with stark reality and thus shattering all his dreams and wishes as constructive either. I can hear you saying, "O.K., faced with a paradox such as this, how am I to proceed in an interaction with this patient? How am I supposed to help reduce the gap between wish and belief, between fact and illusion, without stripping the patient of all hope?" The remainder of this chapter addresses these issues. As a starting point let us look again at some of the philosophical perspectives of hope.

Marcel tells us:

the less life is experienced as a captivity the less the soul will be able to see the shining of that veiled, mysterious light, which we feel sure without any analysis illuminates the very centre of hope's dwelling place (p. 32).

We all know of situations that exemplify this statement. For example, the young man who, when told he has leukemia, begins to see every day, every creature as beautiful and precious, and with hope. Previously he had accepted these things matter-of-factly; almost without thought. What differentiates this young man from another who, given the same diagnosis, falls into despair and unresolved grief? Perhaps it is, as previously mentioned, that while the first young man wishes he were well, he has been helped to believe that he should live each day as fully as he can and for as long as he is able. He views life as a captivity which he continues to strive to overcome. The person who continues to grieve prefers (albeit unconsciously) to turn his anger against himself and others as a part of his refusal to acknowledge the loss of himself as an attachment object. He does not allow himself to experience life in a real sense as a captivity which, in turn, is the stimulus for hope. Rather, he continues in a state of aggressive self-complacency that is often characterized by such attitudes as: "I am sure I am a hopeless case," and, "I doubt if you can do anything for me and, furthermore, I dare you to try!" (Marcel, p. 33).

HOPE VS. OPTIMISM

Marcel also makes a philosophical distinction between hope and optimism (pp. 33–34). The optimistic patient may have a firm conviction that things will turn out for the best, thus again denying the reality of the situation. Delaney-Naumoff notes that denial is one of the essential states of the grief process because it allows the acutely ill individual a respite from the burden of reality at a time when his energies are needed for more critical work such as the work of healing and, in some instances, survival (see Chapter 4). However, if this denial continues beyond the acute phase of illness or disability it can seriously interfere with the acceptance of measures that lead toward optimal health and functioning. To clarify further, Marcel writes:

> When we come down to the final analysis, the optimist, as such, always relies upon an experience which is not drawn from the most intimate and living part of himself, but, on the contrary, is *considered from a sufficient distance* to allow certain contradictions to become alternated or fused into a general harmony . . . there is a pessimism which is the exact counterpart of such optimism. . . . They are like the inside and outside of the same garment (p. 34).

Optimism is equally as much of a problem for the nurse as it is for the patient because it implies a spectator role rather than a true involvement in the interpersonal process of healing. The "optimistic" nurse can distance herself from the reality of what is going on with the patient because, in addition to her spectator role, she also develops the added "virtue" of particularly keen insight. This attitude is often expressed in terms such as: "If you, patient, could see your situation as clearly as I see it, you would have unwavering trust in my judgment and my prescriptions for your problems." This attitude does not promote real engagement on the part of the nurse, the patient, the family, or whoever holds it, with the true nature of the problem.

HOPE AND THE PROCESS OF INVOLVEMENT

Hope, on the other hand, is real and refers to becoming involved in a process. Marcel points out that the concept of "I hope" cannot be interpreted as my being privy to the great secret while all others are viewed as uncomprehending outsiders. Neither can hope be viewed in a materialistic sense, because we have all seen cases where hope has been able to survive when the person is in almost total ruin. Hope cannot exist except where the temptation to despair also exists. "Hope is the act by which this temptation is actively and victoriously overcome" (p. 36).

It seems to me that this aforementioned definition of hope applies equally to nurses and other health workers as it does to patients. For a nurse to become involved with a patient in the process of hoping vs. despair means that the nurse will often share the same feelings being experienced by the patient. When the patient feels hopeful, the nurse will feel hopeful; when the patient approaches despair, the nurse may also despair—not necessarily in the same magnitude, nor in that order. This sharing is the essence of the empathic response that is so much a part of the nurse-patient interaction. Engagement in this process, on the part of the nurse, requires that the nurse receive as much support as she is being expected to give. The profession of nursing must attend to making this kind of support an integral part of one's work role. If nurses cannot expect to receive needed support from their peers and supervisors, then there is no way they can be expected to engage in the kind of process I am speaking of in regard to generating feelings of hope in their patients.

Referring again to Marcel's thesis, we find that in order to understand hope one must understand two distinct attitudes: capitulation and acceptance (pp. 37–38). It has been my experience that clear definitions of these terms are necessary because health workers often seem to attribute the same meaning to both. The first of these attitudes, capitulation, refers to the person who, under the sentence of ill health or disability, goes to pieces and essentially renounces the idea of remaining himself. This person seems to become fascinated by the notion of his own destruction and cannot cope with what has happened in a more productive way. To accept means to keep a firm grip on oneself and to work toward safeguarding one's integrity. Contrary to popular belief, acceptance implies a refusal on the part of the individual to be condemned or to give up and become a useless person in the face of diminishing health. The attitude of acceptance does not imply a denial of what has happened, nor should it be confused with stoicism. The person who accepts his illness or disability is not locked into himself as is the stoic. There is also an element of nonacceptance in the kind of acceptance being discussed, and both the acceptance and nonacceptance components are encompassed in the concept of hope. This kind of nonacceptance does not imply revolt. On the other hand, neither does it imply a tightening or a constricting of oneself into the immovable self-oriented position of the stoic.

We are speaking of hope as encompassing an acceptance of the problem while also continuing with a forward-looking nonacceptance of all the restrictions that the problem is so apt to imply, or restrictions that health workers are so apt to tell the patient about on the chance that the patient has not thought of them himself.

Marcel tells us, "If we introduce the element of patience into nonacceptance, we at once come very much nearer to hope" (p. 39). For the patient and his helpers a significant guideline is, "take your time." This does not mean sloughing off and constantly being late with nursing interventions. Rather, it means that we must begin to understand the personal rhythms (our own, those of patients, family members, and others) and to work with these rhythms rather than to ignore or force them. If one attempts to force the personal rhythms of another, that is, tries to change the regular and recurring patterns of another's psychological and biological patterns or processes, then it becomes less likely that optimum results will occur in spite of otherwise well-intended efforts. Understanding and becoming sensitive to the personal rhythms of another person, as these rhythms relate to our own, can only occur in the context of a relationship in which the patient (or other) becomes meaningful to us and we to them. In supervision with students I frequently find myself telling them to "hang loose" and they will get much further along the way toward reaching their goals than if they allow themselves to become anxious and constricted. The message is, "Hang loose, and *be!*" I frequently surprise myself when I find how much my "vision" improves if I can just relax and spend some time thinking through any problematic situation. Becoming uptight causes functional blindness.

As nurses we should guard against the assumption that we can bend someone else's rhythm to our own by force. Though God knows, we often try. Marcel writes that we must have confidence in a certain process of growth and development:

> To give one's confidence does not merely mean that one makes an act of theoretical acceptance with no idea of intervention, for that would, in fact, be to abandon the other purely and simply to himself. No, to have confidence here seems to mean to embrace this process, in a sense, so that we promote it from within (p. 40).

If this sounds like an ideal state, I suppose in some ways it is. However, there is reality in it, too. The reality is in saying that it is important for the helping person, be it nurse or other, to have a sense of patience and hope in working with the ill and disabled. When we despair of the other person, then we, in essence, have abandoned them. We have communicated that we, too, believe that they are unsalvageable and good for nothing. The attitudes of acceptance, patience, and, ultimately, hope, are difficult to maintain because it is so easy to shift into inactivity or to assume a wait-and-see position as a defense against one's own discouragement.

This brings us to the topics of involvement and risk taking as these affect the practice of nursing. If I am to engage with my patients in a process of grief resolution, of moving from despair to hope, then I must risk the inevitable. I must become involved with this other person, called patient, in the process of safeguarding each of us in terms of our individual integrity. We must work against becoming rigid and viewing the setback of illness as a defeat whereby one or the other of us must relinquish control. We must work together, this patient and I, and I must not stand back like a spectator who thinks that it is only my "Rahs" or "Boos" that will actually turn the tide in this game.

If we look at the process of moving from despair to hope as something that the patient and the nurse share, this does not mean that the nurse must join the patient, in kind, in every play in order for the process to become a success. I am reminded here of an example from psychiatry that seems to illustrate this point. Harry Stack Sullivan (Kvarnes and Parloff, 1976) was discussing the handling of an interaction with a schizophrenic young man who, in a treatment session, had announced that he would like to have genital intimacy with Sullivan. Sullivan stayed with the patient in the process, and he did so without rebuff or without engaging with the patient in the destructive elements of what the patient said he desired. Sullivan merely said to the patient, "Sure I think zonal pleasures are all right, but I am selling expert service and not having a good time" (pp. 216–17). In Sullivan's response there is no disconfirmation of the patient because he wished for something that was contrary to therapeutic goals. There was no shattering of the patient's belief in himself as a person, and there was no flight from the interpersonal process on the part of the helping person. Also, Sullivan appears to do no violence to the personal rhythm of the patient. He meets the patient where he is and gently offers him another direction in which to move, namely, to take advantage of his (Sullivan's) psychiatric expertise.

How does all of this relate to helping patients resolve grief associated with illness or disability? There is always the temptation to join the patient in his despair because we are oriented toward the material aspects of life, and our body is one of our most cherished material possessions. We do not like to get dents in our car or cigarette burns in the sofa cushions. Compared to one's own body or anyone else's body whose imperfections threaten our image of a perfect self, a dent in a car or a burn in the sofa cushion is a trifle.

Here again, the notion of joining in the process with the patient in working through the stages of grief seems the best recommendation to give. Oftentimes instead of joining with the patient in striving for hope, we stand back and observe the patient's grief from a great emotional distance. When we do this the patient becomes more of a possession than a person in need of understanding. And, as with all of our possessions, we do not like to have them reflect poorly on our skills or on our ability to control and manage events. This is so because, as with all possessions, we see them as we need to see them—as extensions of ourselves. This creates a situation that can lead to extreme frustration for the nurse. If individuals cannot control their possessions this speaks poorly for them as owners—if not in the eyes of others, then in their own eyes. That old warning "What will the neighbors think!" operates very effectively in nursing. Our actions are often governed more by what we think the neighbors will think (i.e., our peers and our colleagues) than by what our patients or we think.

The philosophy of Marcel holds that to help another person achieve hope and to liberate him from the despair that so often comes with life-threatening events requires love (pp. 47–49). This is a special kind of love that must, in fact, be reciprocal. It is a love that either through its bond unites me to myself, or unites me to a significant other.

> To love anybody is to expect something from him, something which can neither be defined nor foreseen, it is at the same time in some way to make it possible for him to fulfill this expectation (p. 49).

This statement may seem paradoxical and yet, as Marcel points out, if I expect something from someone I also am in some way giving to that person. If I no longer expect anything from that person, then I have helped to remove his being from him and have set barriers in the way of any creativity or inventiveness that may otherwise have been possible for him (p. 189). This view is supported by Laing and Buber (Watzlawick et al., 1967, pp. 84–87) who infer that in order to love oneself, one must be loved by another, and, to be loved by another increases one's capacity to love oneself. Thus engaging with a patient in the process of grief resolution is an act of love. It is love because we help another person reconfirm his being when we, too, reconfirm it.

DISCONFIRMATION AS CONTRARY TO HOPE

One of the most devastating things we can do to another human being is to engage in a process of disconfirming the other. Watzlawick et al. (1967) note that disconfirmation is different from outright rejection of the other's definition of self. For example, if a newly disabled person says to me, "I am no longer a worthwhile person," I can reject his statement and say through behavior and words, "You are wrong, I will not accept that definition of you." Disconfirmation, on the other hand, implies that we think of the other as being totally incapable of reaching a definition of himself. The staff on rounds who speak about the patient as if he were not there are disconfirming that patient. The clerk in a department store who conducts her sales with a disabled person through his or her able-bodied companion is engaging in an act of disconfirmation. Again quoting from Watzlawick et al., "In other words, while rejection amounts to the message 'You are wrong,' disconfirmation says in effect 'You do not exist.'" (p. 86).

It would be interesting to study how many of the encounters between patients and their helpers smack of disconfirmation. A common example of disconfirmation of another is seen in the way we categorize or stereotype people. Agee refers to stereotyping of the elderly as a practice that erases their individuality (see Chapter 6). The same kind of stereotyping occurs with the physically disabled. They are often viewed as mentally incompetent, asexual beings because their bodies do not function properly. An example of disconfirmation, which vividly stands out in my memory, occurred when I was a patient in a rehabilitation hospital. One day, as I was sitting on the toilet, a volunteer brought a group of visitors through the bathroom. The volunteer threw back the curtain that served as the door of the toilet stall, exposing both me and my wheelchair (the latter of which was slightly more socially acceptable at that moment). Then the volunteer proudly announced to the group of visitors, "This is one of our quadriplegics!" I literally felt as though I was nothing, and as far as meaning anything, I did not. I might just as well have been a resident on monkey island at the zoo. In order to reconfirm that I was indeed somebody, I shouted a few phrases that would have made a longshoreman blush. The volunteer and the visitors retreated while uttering comments about what an ungrateful, uncouth wretch I was. Well, at least "ungrateful and uncouth" constitutes an identity of sorts and one which at that moment I preferred to no identity at all. And then we, as nurses, often wonder why patients fight back and engage in so-called obnoxious behaviors. Too often nurses and other health professionals, like the volunteer in the previous example, see only the effect or outcome and fail to look to themselves for the cause.

THE POSSIBLE, THE IMPROBABLE, AND
THE IMPOSSIBLE

Nursing's responsibility also includes the necessity of assisting patients to look at what is possible and what is not within the scope of their power. Since we do not always know exactly what is possible for some patients who have long-term illnesses or acquired disabilities, we need to be open-minded when discussing options, while at the same time setting limits on those things that are beyond our power. Mrs. C., a nurse who took care of me during the early weeks after I had been pronounced "a complete quadriplegic" and been told that I would never walk again, shared a story with me about her son. It seems that he, too, had been told that he was a quadriplegic and would never walk again. Mrs. C said that her son had exercised every muscle he could while he was on a stryker frame. Even if the best he could do was wiggle a toe, he wiggled it. When it was time to take him off the stryker frame, he walked off! Mrs. C. and I talked about how this was not possible for someone whose spinal cord had been severed, but her son had been misdiagnosed. Since no one had actually visualized my spinal cord yet there seemed to be a fifty-fifty chance that things might not be as bad as they seemed. We also talked about what to expect in the event that the worst proved to be true, that is, that my spinal cord actually was severed (and, I am happy to say that it was not). I have always appreciated being offered the chance to discuss the good possibilities as well as the bad. Somehow it made the bad easier to accept. More importantly, I was helped to hope.

But hope must also have some limits. One should not be unreasonable in encouraging another to believe in something that is known to be impossible. If someone is grieving the loss of a leg, certainly no one would encourage that person to believe that he might grow another one. However, the helping person could assist in working through the grief related to the loss, while at the same time helping the patient look forward to the fact that it is possible to be fitted with a prosthesis. The patient can be helped to realize that he can learn to use the prosthesis almost as well as he could his own leg, or, in some cases, even better.

As a graduate student, I worked with a high school boy who had been born with one normal and one severely deformed leg. For years he had hobbled around on a makeshift extension for his deformed leg. He had even tried to play basketball in gym class. In spite of his efforts to compete, he could not. He frequently fell down or got in the way of the other kids because he could not move as fast as they could. The other kids, he said, laughed at him, ridiculed him, or just told him to go away. His family was very poor and could do no more to provide medical care than what had been accomplished by the time he reached high school. One of his teachers managed to find an agency that was willing to pay for corrective surgery and rehabilitation. Thus he came to the hospital where I was collecting data on long-term orthopedic patients with whom nursing personnel experienced difficulty (Werner, 1959).

The recommendation of the orthopedic surgeon had been to amputate this young man's deformed leg and then fit him with a prosthesis that would match his normal leg. Nurses, doctors, and family members had expected this young man to be thrilled with this plan. Even though he had agreed to the plan, his postsurgical response was one of grieving rather than one of joy. When I first met him he was expressing anger indirectly through passive resistance to measures prescribed to strengthen his stump in preparation for use of his prosthesis. He was referred to me because, by their own admission, the nurses could not tolerate his behavior. He was, for that reason, exactly the type of patient I wanted for my thesis sample.

Talking to this young man was a real eye-opener. Much of his identity, he revealed, was bound up in his deformity. He was the class clown. Although he did not like this role he had worked hard to turn a deficit into a vehicle for acceptance; especially with other kids. Now that he could no longer envision himself as the clown he needed to talk to someone about just who he was. Another problem was that he had no concept of this thing called a prosthesis. He had never known anyone who had one and so he really could not believe that it would work to his advantage. He wished that it would, but without this basis for imagination he could not begin to hope that things would be better than they had been. His stump was smaller than his other thigh at the same level, and so he despaired about that too. He wondered why he should do the exercises when he could not imagine how his stump could possible do the job for which it was intended. Although he had resisted doing the prescribed exercises, had acted silly, and was annoying to the nurses who tried to help him, once he was able to express some of his concerns he participated in treatment in a more meaningful way.

My interactions with this patient consisted of listening to him and sharing with him my feeling that I, too, would be angry if no one bothered to explain things so I could understand and know what to expect. In addition, we worked on some counter-pressure exercises to demonstrate to him just how strong his stump actually was. We talked about how he tended to sell himself short in many areas. One of my nursing goals was to help the patient look realistically at his options and, indeed, to foster in him an increased sense of hope for the future. His beliefs about what he could accomplish changed remarkably in the period of four days in which I had contact with him. I think this is an important part of this story. I had four days in which to work with the patient and I did not spend appreciably more time with him each day than anyone else who was providing nursing contacts. I did, however, have in mind the goal of assessing, intervening, and evaluating the nature of my interactions with the patient, and these interactions took place during the course of providing total nursing care.

The next question is, "What does the nurse do when all evidence points to the fact that the patient has capitulated?" that is, when the patient has given in to despair in spite of all attempts at appropriate nursing intervention. First, we need to distinguish between periods of disappointment and actual despair. Disappointment is a temporary setback that is not incompatible with the concept of hope (Marcel, p. 55). In the course of dealing with long-term illness and disability, everyone has periods when mood is deflated, when things do not go exactly as expected, but this is a part of living as it is with anyone else who has felt disappointment. Disappointment does not mean that the person has forfeited all claim to hope. Despair, on the other hand, is more all-encompassing, it is a total capitulation, it is the abandonment of hope.

With the despairing patient, confrontation may be an important part of the nurse-patient process. The nurse might say, in effect, "You really seem to enjoy making yourself and everyone else suffer." How the nurse would move from that point would depend upon the patient's response to such a statement. If the patient becomes angry and argues that the nurse's perception is incorrect, at least the nurse will have a basis for further discussion at that time. If the patient shows no response and remains mute and withdrawn, other action on the part of the nurse will be necessary.

If the nurse feels comfortable with the discussion, she may be able and willing to pursue highly affective topics. If the nurse does not feel comfortable, but does recognize the seriousness of the problem, she should consult with a psychiatric nurse clinician, a psychiatrist, or other mental health worker and, if necessary, refer the patient to this other professional for help. It is important that all professional staff involved with the patient remain in close communication with each other. This helps to develop continuity in care plans and increases competence among staff dealing with various facets of the patient's problem. In other words, referring a patient to a psychiatric nurse clinician or other health professional does not allow other nurses to abdicate their responsibility for learning as much as they can about working with and enhancing their own process interaction with the patient.

ADDITIONAL NURSING CONSIDERATIONS

Nursings' responsibility in the process of instilling hope is not impossible even though it may not always be easy. The process is replete with paradoxes such as: set limits on unrealistic expectations, but do not kill hope by imposing the restraints of established experience. There just may be a chance that established experience is either inaccurate or incomplete. We see shining examples of this kind of hope in cancer research. Established experience tells us that cancer is a killer. Yet the people who work on cancer research do so on the premise that current knowledge of the disease, while not necessarily inaccurate, is nevertheless incomplete. These researchers defy what seems obvious and known by continuing to look for new solutions. They continue to hope, and along with them, so do we.

This is the attitude that the nurses who work with the chronically ill and disabled are asked to develop. Keep your feet on the ground, while still maintaining a "perhaps" attitude. Perhaps things can change, perhaps all is not lost, perhaps there is something good beyond that which now seems so bad. To say, "Do not be too empirical" in these days when we are feeling a need to validate everything, may seem like blasphemy. But what is wrong with telling a patient something like the following: "According to current evidence this is and this is not now possible for you. However, it wasn't too many years ago that we thought putting a man on the moon was a comic strip fantasy. Nothing is always as it is today." One of the things about hope is that while it cannot see what is going to happen "it affirms it as *if* it saw" (Marcel, p. 62).

Marcel asks if one can hope when the reasons for doing so are insufficient or even completely lacking (p. 64). Why not? When one continues to hope in the face of overwhelming evidence to the contrary, who of us is actually able to say that there are insufficient reasons for hoping? The evidence must be sufficient for the person who continues to hope whether we think so or not. The opposite is also true. There are times when we think the evidence on the side of hope is sufficient, and we do not understand or empathize with the patient who despairs. Obviously the evidence for hope is not sufficient, or does not seem sufficient, for that person at that time.

Hope, then, is the ability on the one hand to transcend what is and to be able to look at the experience as the pledge and first fruits of what is to be (Marcel, p. 67). Hope is the ability to see that the person within a body that has many imperfections is still someone worth knowing, a person who has the right to be. It is reported that when Father Damien was asked how he could tolerate working with lepers, he replied in effect, that they who only see the disease are blind. Anyone with vision would see the person residing within. Nurses need to, and I think often do, strive to see the person within. The rest flows naturally—love, confirmation of being, hope, and the resolution of grief.

REFERENCES

Kvarnes, R. C., and Parloff, G. H., 1976. *A Harry Stack Sullivan case seminar: treatment of a young male schizophrenic.* New York: W. W. Norton and Company, Inc.

Marcel, G. 1962. *Homo viator: introduction to a metaphysic of hope.* (Tr. by Emma Chanfurd.) New York: Harper Torchbooks.

Watzlawick, P.; Beaven, J. H.; and Jackson, D. D. 1967. *Pragmatics of human communication.* New York: W. W. Norton and Company, Inc.

Werner, J. A. 1959. Some factors underlying the behavioral reactions of long-term orthopedic patients with whom nurses experienced difficulty. Unpublished Masters Thesis, The University of Washington, Seattle.

CHAPTER EIGHT

The Burnout Syndrome in Nurses

Irene L. Beland

INTRODUCTION

Two points are considered in this chapter.[1] First, nurses are human beings who have the same needs as other human beings. They respond to need satisfaction or deprivation in ways similar to other human beings who experience similar circumstances. The second point is addressed in the follow-

---

[1] Editor's note: The major portion of this chapter was presented by Irene L. Beland at the Detroit District Annual Meeting and banquet on May 25, 1977. It then appeared as a two-part publication in *News and Views*, November, 1977 and Winter, 1978, 31 and 32. Although the original paper was not intended specifically for nurses who care for individuals with long-term illnesses or disabilities, the points included are certainly most applicable. There are factors involved in the care of individuals with long-term illnesses and disabilities that predispose to the development of the burnout syndrome. For example, some patients fail to improve despite excellent nursing care. For this important reason we are grateful to the author and to *News and Views* of the Detroit District, Michigan Nurses Association, for permission to include this work.

ing questions: What are some of the circumstances causing stress in the practice of nursing? How is this stress manifested, and what can be done to reduce its effects?

In our concentration upon the needs of those we serve, as well as others in the health care system, we often fail to give sufficient attention to the fact that nurses live in the same world as other human beings and have the same needs as these others. We fail to recognize that nurses are affected by the same elements in society as are others. For better or worse, nurses also respond to stress in the same ways as non-nurses respond. However, the nurse "has to grieve in private, smile in public, and praise and receive one's critics" (Gortner, 1977, p. 619).

To emphasize the expectations placed on nurses, I have taken an "advertisement" for traffic controllers at Chicago's O'Hare Airport (Martindale, 1977) and have paraphrased it as an "advertisement for nurses." The advertisement for nurses might read:

> Help wanted. World's busiest hospital seeks nurses skilled in all areas of human disaster. Knowledge of sophisticated machines including the computer helpful. Work in an unusually stimulating and high-intensity environment. Must be able to cope with patients and their relatives as well as physicians and administrators in all states of consciousness and emotion. Must be able to project a warm, friendly demeanor no matter what the demands nor how great the provocation. Expected to infer the state of the patient from incomplete data and to act appropriately. That is, to institute emergency measures, call the physician or supervisor, or watch and wait for further developments. When errors occur, will, of course, assume full responsibility irrespective of who really is responsible, or, of the number of people involved. No degree required. Hospital Administration will subsidize three quarter credits per term. Salary com-

mensurate with the fact that the hospital is a nonprofit agency.

Recently, nurses who read *One Flew Over the Cuckoo's Nest* (Kesey, 1962) or saw the movie have written with less than great sympathy for Nurse Ratched. What these critics fail to realize is that Nurse Ratched was reacting to a situation in a way that insured her emotional survival. This is not meant to imply that this was the only reaction available to her as there are always other alternatives. But apparently Nurse Ratched needed support which she did not seek or receive in order to see what these other alternatives might have been. Further, Nurse Ratched was not unique in her reactions.

That nurses are not alone in their reactions to stressful situations is demonstrated in a study by Dr. Christina Maslach of the University of California (1976). Dr. Maslach studied some 200 persons—doctors (including psychiatrists), poverty lawyers, child care workers, mental health nurses, and policemen. All were found to have difficulty coping with the emotional stress from intimate involvement with troubled human beings. Maslach called the condition that resulted "burnout." Some law enforcement groups call this same configuration of behaviors the "John Wayne Syndrome."

HUMAN NEEDS

Needs and the ability to meet one's needs are important for the nurse practitioner. In this chapter the term *needs* is defined as a necessity or requirement which, if not supplied, leads to some change in behavior. If the deprivation is severe it can lead to sickness or even death.

The following generalizations are being made about needs: (1) Needs may be material or nonmaterial. Oxygen is a material substance; love is nonmaterial. (2) Whatever the need, a continued supply is necessary. (3) Needs are organized into a hierarchy with basic or survival needs generally taking precedence over higher needs. (4) There are mechanisms for supplying needs. The more important the need is for survival the more mechanisms there are to provide supply. (5) There are warning signals (signs and symptoms) that indicate that needs are or are not being met. When needs are not met the symptoms or signals only indicate that something is wrong, and not what is wrong. (6) The satisfaction of one need is influenced by and influences the satisfaction of other needs. (7) The anatomical, physiological, and emotional state of a person affects his ability to tolerate the frustration of a need. (8) Supply may be inadequate, adequate, or excessive. Depending upon the degree, either a deficiency or an excess in supply may have damaging effects (Maslow, 1954).

Physiological needs are the requirements that cells have if they are to carry on their activities. These requirements are not unique to human beings, but are the needs of all living things—plants and animals. These physiological needs generally take precedence over higher needs.

Next in the hierarchy are safety needs. Psychologists often emphasize the importance of the *feeling* of safety. However, physical safety is also important. Many hospital policies are directed toward the physical safety of patients, and some policies are also oriented toward the maintenance of physical safety for nurses. These include infection control, devices and procedures to reduce the strain on nurses' backs, as well as the protection of nurses from assaultive patients.

In the past little attention has been focused on the importance of the feeling of safety in patients and nurses within the actual treatment settings. There is a need for individualization of care because what one person experiences as a threat to personal safety cannot necessarily be generalized to all persons, or even to the same person in varying states of physical or emotional health. If we define any need as a constant, we are in danger of then defining any deviation from that constant as a personality problem or pathological behavior. Maslow (1962) states:

Clearly what will be called personality problems depends on who is doing the calling. . . . It seems quite clear that personality problems may be loud protests against the crushing of one's psychological bones, or one's true inner nature (p. 7).

Measures taken to increase the patient's feeling that he can depend upon the nursing staff to meet his needs (psychological and physical) may well decrease the patient's demands, and, in turn, increase nurses' satisfaction with their profession.

Among the higher needs are the nonmaterial or psychological needs: needs for love, self-esteem, and self-actualization (Maslow, 1954). The same generalizations can be made about psychological needs as were made for physical needs. That is, everyone has them. As with the physiological or lower order needs, the supply may be insufficient, too great, or optimum. Further, the supply must be replenished or the pitcher runs dry. One further point, each individual has to make appropriate efforts to supply his own needs or to seek help from others as necessary. "You more than anyone else in your world determines the state of your emotions. If someone offends or hurts or disappoints you, it is because you have given him the power to do so" (Olson, 1974, p. 23).

What are love needs as these relate to professional life? These include a feeling of acceptance by peers, recognition that one is an accepted member of a group, that one is an essential part of the operation, giving and receiving friendship, and having a mutually respecting and trusting relationship with others.

A cohesive work group is generally more effective than the same number of people working separately because the group provides an adequate referent or anchor point for its members. That is, the members come to know the norms of the group and how these affect each member's need requirements. Group norms tell the individuals what is expected and what is not, as well as what is acceptable and what is not. This provides the members with cues as to how the group can and will meet their needs; it also provides a sense of security and room for creativity among the members.

Some management practices prevent the development of an espirit de corps which facilitates working relationships because management believes that a cohesive group may frustrate rather than facilitate organizational objectives. Among these practices is the dealing out of nursing personnel as if they are cards. The nurse seldom is certain where she will be working or with whom. Opportunities to develop trust in or to obtain support from co-workers is nil. Certain nurses may like the challenge of working on a new unit each day, but this practice makes it difficult to develop the feeling that one is truly a part of a health care team, the members of which have common objectives. On the other hand, one cannot be held responsible for much when the excuse "I don't work here regularly" has considerable validity. Most nurses, however, find it difficult to gain satisfaction from the knowledge that they are an important part of the health care system when they are moved hither and yon. Without consistency in membership on the unit team, it is also impossible to develop support systems for nurses.

Transferring individuals from one nursing unit to another also reduces the opportunity for developing real knowledge and expertness in an area. Even the monthly rotation, justified on the basis of "keeping nurses flexible" may interfere with the development of competence, with the feeling that one has a significant contribution to make and is respected for it, and with the development of a commitment to the norms of a particular group.

Among the most important psychological needs of people are the esteem needs. Esteem needs include the need to experience positive attitudes and behaviors of others toward us—attitudes that reflect love and respect. From this an individual learns to esteem himself without reservation or fear (McKeachie & Doyle, 1966, p. 221). Esteem can be defined as self-confidence, a good opinion of one's self, or approval and respect for oneself. In one of his columns, Sidney J. Harris, a syndicated columnist, wrote that "esteem is the secret opinion of yourself, whether it is too high, too low, arrogant or ashamed—it is reflected not only in the eye, but also in all that proceeds from eye-to-eye contact: in posture, gesture, tone and gait. Phonies are not those who lie to others, but to themselves."

Each of you brought to nursing your own opinion of yourself. You may have shared portions of this opinion with others, but other parts you may have hidden, more or less, even from yourself. Any or all dimensions of one's personal assessment may be true, partly true, or false. The important thing is that these dimensions constitute your picture of yourself, or your self-concept, and have a significant effect upon your approach to life and what you accomplish. When esteem needs are satisfied, then, theoretically, one can move on to more self-actualizing motives—competence, curiosity, achievement, and organization (McKeachie and Doyle, 1966, p. 221).

When you entered nursing, in addition to bringing with you your self-esteem or self-confidence, you also brought with you techniques for supplying your self-esteem or repairing damage to it. Whatever its state, in nursing there are many potential threats to self-esteem. Some of these derive from the real and/or perceived nature of relationships: man-woman; doctor-nurse; supervisor-supervisee; pateint-nurse; giving-receiving; will I make it?—won't I? and so on. Esteem, or the lack of it, for nursing also derives from the status position of the profession as compared to medicine, psychology, social work and so forth, as well as from the status position of women in our society and in the health care professions.

Evidence of lack of self-esteem, self-confidence, or respect for oneself or the nursing profession is evidenced in statements such as, "I'm *only* a student nurse" or "I'm *only* a nurse." I am of the opinion that the excessive obsession with the question "What is nursing?" is also evidence of excessive concern with what others think of our professional behavior and importance.

POWER MOTIVES AND NEEDS

The basis upon which nurses make the previously mentioned comparisons and arrive at what are often negative conclusions about their own self-worth needs considerable attention in the education and practice domains of nursing. Closely akin to the esteem motive, it seems to me, is the power motive that McClelland defines as, "a thought about someone *having impact*" (1975, p. 7). McClelland indicates that the difficulty in drawing conclusions from the masses of data concerning male-female behavior results from the tendency of psychologists to regard male behavior as the norm and female behavior as a deviation from the norm. One of the main dimensions on which women score high is in the interdependence category. Because of this, women may require more supportive relationships, not because they are dependent or neurotic, but because they are women. McClelland states, "Since interpersonal relationships are more important for women, therefore, it is more worrying, more necessary to make an adjustment when someone disapproves. The men may not notice or care" (pp. 81–86).

Among professional women with a high power motive, not all assume masculine, assertive characteristics, although some do and with considerable ease and comfort. What usually happens according to McClelland is that women with a high power motive want to build up resources, especially their physical-material resources, so that they have more to share; their scores on the interdependence dimension are usually higher than for women who score lower on power motivation. The women with high power motivation also tend to join more organizations where control is important. Another interesting observation made by McClelland is that women who develop a high power motive are helped by it to move to higher stages of maturity. Evidence indicates that in men a high power motive tends to hinder their movement toward higher stages of maturity (pp. 94–96).

Understanding this interdependence dimension and the giving-sharing tendency among power motivated women becomes extremely important in nursing. "Women are concerned with the context; men are forever trying to ignore it for the sake of something they can abstract from it" (McClelland, p. 89). What this statement implies in the health professions is that doctors (mostly male) and nurses (mostly female) come at the same problem from their different and unique perspectives. To expect sameness is to breed frustration.

Another point is that when looking at nursing as a predominantly female profession, then the interdependence dimension of its members requires a consistent feedback system in order to maintain maximum effectiveness. Without feedback and support one does not need much imagination to envision burnout occurring rather quickly. On the other hand, there is nothing so sacred about female interdependence to preclude that some female nurses have been socialized differently and are naturally more assertive and independent. These nurses also require understanding and support because if society dictates that one *must* be interdependent, then woe be unto the nurse (male or female) who goes against this stereotype (McClelland, pp. 92–93).

Returning now to self-esteem per se, we can ask, "What are its underpinnings?" These include knowledge (and knowledge is for any nurse who is willing to work for it; competence, which continues to improve; and, independence, with the ability also to be interdependent and dependent. This means that the nurse must have some control over working conditions and to be able to work with others, to have prestige and status, to be able to gain satisfaction from a job well done, to continue to grow and renew herself, to have an income sufficient to provide for her needs, and also to be able to provide for her old age. This income should be comparable to that of others who have similar preparation and responsibilities.

Self-actualization—what is it? Briefly, self-actualization is a state of becoming, a state which some question whether it exists or is ever fully achieved. Self-actualization does not mean self-centeredness. Rather, it means that a person recognizes and develops his talents. Maslow writes that self-actualization stresses "full humanizing," and that self-actualized people are altruistic, social, dedicated, and self-transcending (1962, p. iii). Because the self-actualized person has a commitment to excellence, the person continues to learn and grow. This implies too that she selects a field on the basis of her talents and interests, and not just on the basis of the salary or power inherent in the position. To emphasize this point, I quote John Gardner:

> An excellent plumber is infinitely more admirable than an incompetent philosopher. The society that scorns excellence in plumbing because plumbing is a humble activity and tolerates shoddiness in philosophy because it is an exalted activity will have neither good plumbing nor good philosophy. Neither its pipes nor its theories will hold water (1961, p. 86).

Although it would be possible to further expand on the concept of needs, suffice it to say that unless a nurse is able to meet her needs in healthy ways she will have difficulty in meeting the needs of patients or clients. I am reminded of a sign I saw in front of a real estate office that said, "We can't do business from an empty wagon."

DETACHMENT VS. DEHUMANIZATION

Other concepts that are useful in understanding the burn-out syndrome and the behaviors that occur as a result are those of detachment and dehumanization. Detachment is a process whereby one person separates himself from another and is distinguished from dehumanization where the one person divests the other of his human qualities. It is interesting to note that when Maslach (Coakley, 1977) asked the subjects in her study if they tended to dehumanize their clients or patients, they all said no. When she asked them if they sometimes tried to detach themselves from their clients or patients, these same subjects said yes. The tendency to detach themselves or hold themselves aloof from patients or clients was true of all subjects in this study.

When a nurse detaches herself from a patient she emotionally or physically separates herself from him. This detachment can be slight. That is, the nurse gains just enough emotional distance from the patient to evaluate the situation from a position of greater objectivity in order to more realistically plan care. This level of detachment does not mean that the nurse is not involved with the patient. Quite the contrary. Emotional involvement on the part of the nurse with the patient may be an essential precursor of therapeutic distancing or detachment. This level of detachment is a schooled or learned process that should become part of each nurse's repertoire of abstract skills. On the other hand, detachment can be profound. That is, there can be so much emotional distancing on the part of the nurse that she begins to function as an automaton without feeling or evident concern for the needs of patients. While a slight degree of detachment is essential at times in most nurse-patient situations, severe or profound detachment, if it is essentially job related, spells burnout.

When the nurse dehumanizes the patient she thinks of the patient as an animal (e.g., a pig or a rat) or makes some other demeaning comparison. There is a fine line separating detachment and dehumanization. Detachment is a response that enables the individual to cope with a continuing high level stressful environment. Dehumanization is the possible result of detachment but goes beyond emotional and physical separation to contempt.

REASONABLE INVOLVEMENT IN NURSING PRACTICE

The following point is missed by some nurse writers who urge nurses to be more expressive of their emotions with patients—to "become *involved!*" Continued high level involvement is exhausting. In defense of one's ego one needs to be able to shut off this investment and to open it up again when needed. One psychiatric nurse, who works as a psychotherapist, states that she "psyches herself up" for each patient and then gives the patient her undivided attention for the period of time he has contracted for. She is able to close off her involvement at other times of her life and to engage in other, self-fulfilling activities. Before randomly prescribing expressing one's emotions with patients, more attention should be given to what patients need and want and also to ways of protecting and restoring one's own emotional balance. The nurse must meet her own needs in ways that enable her to identify the patient's problems and to meet them in a caring or concerned way. The patient has enough problems without being burdened by inappropriate expressions of the nurse's emotions.

It is well to remember a point made by Toffler in *Future Shock* (1970) about involvement. He asserts that "any relationship implies mutual demands and expectations. The more intimately involved a relationship, the greater the pressure the parties exert on one another to fulfill these expectations" (p. 98). In other words, when one becomes involved with a patient, one expects the patient to behave in a certain way, and the patient has certain expectations in return. Unless these expectations are met, one or both participants in the interaction will suffer disappointment. For both patient and nurse this means that the boundaries of the relationship need to be clearly defined, or, as Toffler's work suggests, one needs to be clear about the number and kinds of modules that belong in a particular relationship. For example, a usual relationship with the person who delivers the mail does not bring in modules relating to that person's home life, religion, or socioeconomic status. There is one module in this relationship and it defines the relationship only in terms of whether or not mail is delivered on time and in good condition (p. 98).

Another variable to be considered in determining the degree to which a nurse can or should become involved with a patient is the time or duration of the relationship. If present trends continue, the length of a patient's stay in the hospital often will be short—admittance in the morning and discharge in the afternoon. Under these circumstances the nurse-patient relationship is likely to be superficial and its boundaries clearly defined. In addition to these brief, superficial relationships, however, there are those involving long-term patients which are multifaceted and often become intimate and intense. In medium- or long-term relationships where some degree of emotional involvement on the part of the nurse and patient can be expected, termination of these relationships becomes a problem worthy of our concern. In most people separation increases anxiety. For the individual nurse this means that she needs to be helped to understand her feelings about termination or she will avoid reasonable involvement or become detached and callous. If she cannot understand and deal with her own and the patient's feelings generated by separation, the price of emotional expenditure, for her, becomes too great.

MANIFESTATIONS OF BURNOUT

What evidence indicates that the nurse is not adequately meeting her needs? One possibility is that she shows signs of developing the burnout or the "Ratched" syndrome. The signs and symptoms of burnout or the "Ratched" syndrome are as follows:

1. Using techniques to lessen anxiety and/or to place the patient at a distance. For example, the nurse uses terms for people such as "coronary," "Doctor So-and-So's physical," "the bath in 206," "the poor," "a haircut," "an animal," or she begins describing a stressful event as precisely and as scientifically as possible. Other techniques include the use of jargon, intellectualizing about a situation, or joking or laughing about a stressful event. We all do all of these things on occasion. It is only when these behaviors become the predominating pattern for the nurse that one must think of the possibility of burnout. Maslach cites the example of the M.A.S.H. surgeons telling sick jokes and flirting with the nurses as ways of handling extreme stress in the operating room (p. 19). More will be said later about the use of laughter as an appropriate and common tension reliever. Sometimes I wonder if any of us have learned to laugh enough.

2. Withdrawing or spending less time with patients, or withdrawing to another field. Often nurses escape to a branch of nursing that requires less personal involvement with patients because they cannot cope with tension which the nurse-patient relationship produces in them. As a temporary measure they may escape to the linen closet or the utility room. If the stress from direct patient contact is severe, the nurse may escape to nursing education, research, or administration, or she may elect an entirely different field of endeavor. There is nothing wrong with any of these moves if they truly are solutions. However, if the nurse runs to these other areas and just carries the conflicts along, she has done a disservice to herself because nothing has been resolved. Periodically we all probably think about leaving nursing. I wonder how many times I have talked myself out of raising cows and cabbages!

Nurses are like other human beings, as well as other animals, in so far as they withdraw from painful situations. Either that or they are likely to become obnoxiously aggressive and controlling.

Socializing almost exclusively with other nurses and rehashing and rehashing the work situation is also symptomatic of burnout. There may also be excessive absences from work and/or a refusal to accept certain assignments. Some nurses who have not quite reached the point of burnout may find that they have an overwhelming emotional involvement with the patient and his situation. An excessive degree of involvement results in the nurse being unable to evaluate the patient's needs and to meet these in constructive ways. Indeed, the nurse's feeling of being overwhelmed emotionally does not necessarily mean that she spends more time with the patient, but that she may engage in excessive behind-the-scenes rumination about the patient's plight. Thus, these attempts to withdraw from a painful situation may indicate that the nurse needs supportive intervention in order to cope with the stresses she feels in the work situation.

3. Developing chronic illnesses as a way of coping with stress. Among the traffic controllers at O'Hare and other busy airports, hypertension is four times more common and occurs at an earlier age than in other, less busy airports. At O'Hare, nearly two-thirds of the ninety-four traffic controllers

have peptic ulcers or show signs of developing them (Martindale, p. 72). How does the incidence of these and other disorders in nurses compare with the general population? We don't
know, but this certainly is a topic for research. Hefferin and
Hill (1976), in an analysis of work-related injuries in nursing,
stated that hospitals have a higher incidence of on-the-job
injuries than do many industries and that nursing personnel
have proportionately higher injury rates and lose more work
days than personnel in other departments (p. 924). These
authors did not use length of patient stay or the chronicity of
illness as variables, but it would be interesting to see if the
difficulty of the patients cared for and the amount of gratification nurses receive correlates significantly with the number
of work-related injuries or the rate of absenteeism among
nurses. Hefferin and Hill's data indicated that the majority of
injuries occurring in nursing personnel could have been prevented fairly easily (p. 926). This information makes one
wonder how much the nurses may have emotionally dis-
associated themselves from their task and have, as a result,
become less attentive to potential sources of injury. The result, of course, would be a legitimate reason for absence from
work—a respite from a stressful situation.

Other physical symptoms reported by Martindale and
Maslach as indicators of the burnout syndrome are: insomnia,
loss of appetite, anxiety, instability, and sexual dysfunction,
as well as chain smoking, over-eating, and so forth. Recently
there has been increased concern in nursing and medical
centers about the number of nurses and physicians who are
alcohol and drug abusers.

4. **Other factors identified in burnout.** Pines and Maslach
(1977), in a study of professionals working in psychiatric
settings, found that the severity of the patient's illness was,
indeed, a significant factor in the development of burnout
among these personnel. The more chronic and intractable the
patients' conditions were perceived to be, the more time staff

spent in administrative duties or the more often they recommended pharmacological intervention rather than other forms of intervention requiring longer periods of direct contact with patients (p. 7). In addition to the patient chronicity variable, Pines and Maslach found that the incidence of burnout was also positively correlated with: (1) institutional variables or work conditions, (2) large patient-to-staff ratio, (3) poor work relationships, (4) poor staff/patient relations, (5) increasing numbers of staff meetings that focused on job-oriented rather than patient-oriented goals, (6) few sanctioned timeouts, and (7) long work hours, just to name a few.

In areas such as rehabilitation or oncology, where nurse-patient relationships may be long term, it would seem that these factors are vitally important concerns for nursing administration as well as for the individual nurse. Recently the concept of the nurse as a survivor—especially in areas such as oncology—has received attention (Millerd, 1977). Little has been done, however, to study survivor effects in nurses as a factor related to the broader burnout syndrome. Pines and Maslach did not identify grief or survivor reactions among psychiatric professionals. This seems reasonable since these professionals do not deal with a population of patients where a significant number are in the terminal phase of their lives—where death is constantly anticipated if not an actuality.

MEASURES TO PREVENT BURNOUT

As with other disorders, prevention is preferred to cure. If the nurse or others recognize that high level emotional stress results in increasing tension, then tension-relieving strategies can be introduced before the burnout syndrome begins or while it is still in its early phase. The fact that there is such a syndrome must be accepted. Each nurse is affected by the woes of others and her responses ensure her emotional survival. Just as one person can walk up more flights of stairs than another without signs of respiratory distress, some nurses can cope with an emotionally charged environment for longer periods without showing signs of emotional distress. Each of us, however, has a threshold beyond which we cannot go without reacting in some way.

In a review of motivational theory, Ann Marriner (1976, p. 63) makes the following recommendation, which, if carried out, should be useful in preventing the burnout syndrome. According to Marriner, talents and interests should be considered in assigning jobs. Personnel should be encouraged to contribute to decisions, goals, and plans. All suggestions should be treated with courtesy and respect. Too often suggestions from those lower in the nursing hierarchy are treated as threats to the "holy writ." Perhaps there should be a system of rewards for persons who make usable suggestions. Recently, I read in a newspaper that a man from General Motors had, over the years, been awarded more than one hundred thousand dollars for his suggestions. A practice of rewarding suggestions should encourage both the offering and the accepting of them.

Workloads should be reasonable. Maslach indicates, and most of us would agree, that burnout is inevitable when a professional person has to care for too many people. This results in a higher and higher emotional overload. Similar to an electrical overload, the worker blows a fuse. In evaluating the size of the workload, the needs of each patient must be considered. Not only the number of patients, but the number of hours a nurse must spend meeting each patient's needs should be evaluated. Maslach, for example, found that nurse administrators could work longer hours than nurses working in direct contact with patients, such as those giving direct care to children, without evidence of emotional overload (p. 18).

Hutchins and Cleveland (1978) reported on a staffing pattern for hospital nurses that has proven effective in preventing the symptoms of burnout. These authors refer to this staffing pattern as the 7–70 plan. That is, nurses work a 10-hour day for seven consecutive days followed by seven consecutive days off. Because of the shift overlap provided for in this pattern, one nurse stated, "I like the shift overlap. I go to lunch, take my full half-hour and relax because I know my patients are well cared for. And I don't go home with the feeling that I've been rushed into forgetting something" (p. 233).

Another interesting finding presented by Hutchins and Cleveland is that with the 7–70 plan, because most patients are in the hospital for shorter periods of time, assignments can be made so there is a high probability that the patient will have the same nursing personnel throughout his entire hospital stay. Sick time for staff nurses under this plan is less than half of the estimate for other nursing personnel in the area. The turnover rate with 7–70 is 9 to 10 percent annually as opposed to 25 percent for agencies using traditional 5–40 staffing patterns. After five years, 32 of the original 50 RN's hired when the hospital was opened were still on staff. These 32 strongly endorsed this innovative plan, a plan which apparently not only prevents burnout to a great extent, but also meets with the approval of patients and physicians as well (pp. 230–33).

Other considerations to prevent burnout include specific patient assignments. Nursing personnel should not be sentenced to work with difficult patients. In other words, the nurse should not have to feel trapped. The nurse should, for the sake of patients as well as herself, be able to tell the head nurse or supervisor "I can't cope with him or her." Generally, given the opportunity to discuss the problems she is having in the nurse-patient relationship and given the support of nursing colleagues, the nurse will be able to continue in the relationship. Another technique that is useful is for the group who care for the patient(s) to identify the problems, discuss the nature of the problems, make a plan for problem resolution, and then *carry out the plan,* making modifications as appropriate. Too often a problem is identified but the process stops at this point. Unless problem solving is carried through to a point of making, implementing, and evaluating the effectiveness of a plan, the feeling of hopelessness is intensified rather than relieved.

Sometimes the most effective plan of action is to relieve the tension in the nursing staff itself. Klagsburn (1977), in a chapter entitled, "Cancer, Emotions, and Nurses," gives a detailed account of working to resolve the strain that patients in a cancer research unit placed on the nursing and medical staff. The patients were viewed by the staff as walking dead. "Since, 'one should not speak ill of the dead,' the staff felt constrained to keep their feelings about the patients to themselves" (p. 251). However, the staff were angry and feeling guilty for having angry feelings. The end result was a covert rejection of patients' emotional needs, and power struggles between patients and staff ensued. Using a nonthreatening exploratory group technique with the nurses, Klagburn (a psychiatrist) was able to help the nurses gain a clearer understanding of the doctors' need for distance and their own central role in the care of patients. "The exciting part of the meeting was that for the first time the nurses seemed to be able to accept the emotional burden of patients without expecting to be supported by the doctors"—a dimension of role distinction that had previously been unclear to the nurses (p. 255). Through the support gained from subsequent meetings, the nurses realigned their view of patients along with their expectations of them. After many weeks of group meetings there evolved an entirely new ward culture— one that clearly demonstrated greater mutual respect on the part of both patients and nurses. Patients were no longer seen as the "walking dead" but as human beings with varying degrees of capability to contribute to the ward milieu. As morale on the ward improved, the doctors also became interested and involved in the day-to-day events (pp. 252–262).

Thus tension-relieving strategies should be encouraged. Maslach tells of psychiatric nurses who utilize the technique of assigning nurses to spend a day charting. The old escape to cleaning the utility room or straightening out the linen closet probably made more sense than it was credited with. In another instance, nurses in an intensive care unit were given an extra half-day off after having many patients die in a short period of time. In one psychiatric setting personnel were given seven mental health days per year. For example, a staff nurse could say to the head nurse, "I *really* need to take a mental health day tomorrow." This practice gave the head nurse an opportunity to discuss the stresses of work with the staff nurse. It also gave the staff nurse the feeling that she had a legitimate right to a day off without feeling guilty about having to call in sick.

There should be a kind of crisis intervention therapy available to nurses and others who work in the health care field. Martindale relates that crisis intervention or preventive psychiatry has been recommended for the air traffic controllers at Chicago's O'Hare Airport, using the rationale that burnout in its early stages can be turned around with appropriate available help (p. 72). I see no reason why crisis intervention for nurses would not be an appropriate role for a Master's prepared psychiatric–mental health nurse clinician. Oftentimes nurses discuss their problems in an informal way when they get together for lunch or in the dressing room. One of the failures in this method is that the circumstances under which discussion occurs demands no commitment for follow-through or examination of personal motivations. As a result, these unstructured, informal discussions may reinforce the nurse's feeling of helplessness within the system and actually contribute to the burnout syndrome.

There need to be stronger support systems for nurses within agencies where they work. This includes formal opportunities for planning and evaluating patient care, for the discussion of problems that moves beyond the level of catharsis to the level of understanding the contributing factors as well as the possible outcomes. In addition, each nurse needs to develop her own support system, or, as Gortner (1977) calls them, "strategies for survival in the practice world." Gortner's six strategies for survival are briefly summarized as follows: (1) competence, (2) knowledge of the organization, (3) mastery of the art of the possible, (4) taking advantage of opportunities to do more, (5) recognition of the fact that few problems are original, so there must be a solution somewhere, and (6) building and using one's own support systems (p. 618).

Gortner also stresses the value of non job-related activities—hobbies, interest in the creative arts, and so on. I also think that learning to relax completely, if only for five or ten minutes at a time, can reduce one's tension and function to give one a brighter outlook both for self and for others. On the front page of *National Observer* (March 12, 1977) there appeared a discussion by psychologists regarding what they can do to assist people to live better lives. The headline is, "Wanta be happy? Don't try so hard." The article points out that there is a difference between optimize and maximize. We sometimes forget that if some is good, more may not be better. Furthermore, what is optimal for one person may not be for another. It is important that you get to know yourself and what coping methods work best for you. These may be different coping methods than those used by Mary Smith or Betty Brown. This is to be expected because even though we are all human, we each have learned to live with our humanness in our own unique ways.

Humor is a useful tension reliever when used appropriately. The use of laughter or humor in serious plays and novels is a commonly used tension-relieving technique. Shakespeare was a master of this technique. The physically disabled often engage each other in a kind of "gallows humor" that some of their able-bodied friends find disconcerting. For example, to hear one paraplegic tell another to "shake a leg" instead of saying "hurry up" may leave both of them laughing. By-standers often think such behavior is in bad taste, but what they do not understand is that this kind of humor not only relieves tension for the two paraplegics, it also helps to establish the boundary or "We-ness" of who is in and who is out of their group. Olson (1974) writes, "Laughter is such a marvelous tool to help us hang loose." Referring to his psychotherapeutic techniques, he states, "I use laughter quite a bit as a healing force." At another point Olson says:

> I know sometimes we get so uptight with our own self-worth and importance that perhaps it does us good to go into the bathroom and shut the door, look in the mirror and contemplate God's good sense of humor in creating us.

He goes on to say that we have become experts in building catastrophes out of small things and that many of us are always angry and uptight. Our tendency is to get upset at things we can't change and often not upset enough about things we can change (pp. 72–74). This seems an interesting philosophy and well worth a few moments of our attention.

SUMMARY

Nurses are human beings with all of the strengths and weaknesses of others. Despite some limited preparation in how to cope with situations characterized by high-level stress, nurses, like others who work with people in trouble, have their limits. Whether we call the result the "Ratched," "John Wayne," or the "burnout" syndrome is immaterial. Although the syndrome is not unique to nurses, it needs to be studied in nursing populations. Methods for prevention—or, if need be, treatment—need to be identified and made available so that patients can be better served and nurses can gain increased job satisfaction. As noted in the article by Hutchins and Cleveland, when attention is paid to methods that increase job satisfaction, the result is greater staying power and commitment to nursing as a profession.

One last point, recently a nurse educator and a social worker, on separate occasions, said to me that nurses should stop saying what a lousy job nurses do and, instead, start saying what we do well. We are, after all, the backbone of health and sickness care.

REFERENCES

Coakley, M. Burnout. *Detroit Free Press,* January 3, 1977.

Gardner, J. W. 1961. *Excellence* New York: Harper and Brothers.

Gortner, S. R. 1977. Strategies for survival in the practice world. *American Journal of Nursing* 77:618-19.

Hefferin, E. A., and Hill, B. J. 1976. Analyzing nursing's work related injuries. *American Journal of Nursing* 76: 924-27.

Hutchins, C., and Cleveland, R. 1978. For staff nurses and patients—the 7-70 plan. *American Journal of Nursing* 78: 230-33.

Kesey, K. 1962. *One flew over the cuckoo's nest.* New York: A Signet Book from New American Library.

Klagsburn, S. C. 1977. Cancer, emotions, and nurses. In *Coping with physical illness,* ed. R. H. Moos. New York: Plenum Medical Book Company.

Marriner, A. 1976. Motivation of personnel. *Supervisor Nurse* 7:60-63.

Martindale, D. 1977. Sweaty palms in the control tower. *Psychology Today* 10:70-75.

Maslach, C. 1976. Burned-out. *Human Behavior* 5:16-22.

Maslow, A. H. 1954. *Motivation and personality.* New York: Harper and Brothers.

———. 1962. *Toward a psychology of being.* Princeton, NJ: D. Van Nostrand Company, Inc., An Insight Book.

McClelland, D. C. 1975. *Power: the inner experience.* New York: Irvington Publishers, Inc.

McKeachie, W. J., and Doye, C. L. 1966. *Psychology.* Reading, Mass.: Addison-Wesley Publishing Company, Inc.

Millerd, E. J. 1977. Health professionals as survivors. *JPN and Mental Health Services,* April, 33–37.

Olson, K. 1974. *The art of hanging loose in an uptight world.* Greenwich, Conn.: A Fawcett-Crest Book, Fawcett Publications, Inc.

Pines, A., and Maslach, C. 1977. Detached concern and burnout in mental health professions. Paper presented at the Second Annual National Conference on Child Abuse and Neglect, 17–20 April 1977, at Houston, Texas.

Toffler, A. 1970. *Future shock.* New York: Bantam Books.

Wanta be happy? Don't try so hard. *National Observer,* March 12, 1977.

Index

of certain choices. An important aim for people undergoing chronic stress is to find some pattern or meaning for their existence. Anticipatory mourning may be evidenced here, that is, the beginning of the grief work prior to the actual loss. Often this is a difficult theme for nurses to allow because it triggers their own fears of loss. But, it is highly important that the patient be allowed this expression.

A helpful framework for the nurse to use is to identify previous personality and adaptive patterns the elderly person used and thus avoid jumping to conclusions about altering long-enduring adjustment patterns just because these do not measure up to the nurse's expectations. The major focus for intervention is on those aspects of disturbed behavior which evidence an unintegrated personality, or, toward those aspects of the environment which do not facilitate optimal functioning and life satisfaction.

The main thing I would like to stress about dealing with grieving in the elderly is *not* to stifle it. As painful as it might be for nurses and family members, elderly patients need support in experiencing and expressing grief rather than help in escaping from it. An elderly man in a nursing home sought his family's aid in getting out. In truth, he did not really need to be there since he was self-sufficient and in no physical distress, but none of his immediate family wanted him. Stepchildren had offered him a home but this was some distance from his long-time residential area. One day he asked his stepchildren to drive him to visit a number of old friends and neighbors. One-by-one he asked each of them if they would take him in as a boarder or rent him a small cottage. One-by-one they apologetically came up with reasons, excuses, and rationalizations why they could not do so. The pain and despair he felt was mirrored in his eyes, but he retained some sense of dignity since he knew he had one last option. This final attempt to gain acceptance and control was something he had to do even though it resulted in depression. To sit by and allow him to do this was one of the most difficult and painful experiences I have had. It would have been infinitely easier to have dissuaded him from this pilgrimage or to have refused to drive him. But some grief must be experienced, shared, and borne. One must be open to that, too, if one is to be open to life.

We must not stifle the grieving of our patients. How they manage it is ultimately dependent upon what resources they have and upon what adaptive patterns they bring into the situation. We cannot prevent them from entering the process of grief in order to protect ourselves against the pain. So too with depression. The nurse might focus with the elderly on esteem-building activities: the restoration of some sense of mastery or control over their lives, the restoration of significant memorabilia or objects, or simply human contact— lending an ear to their feelings. In order for individuals to "come up" from depression they need someone to be there—to supportively allow them to experience and express their feelings. It is esteem building to know that another person cares enough about you to be with you during painful periods. These activities can serve to elevate self-esteem and where there is a high level of self-esteem there is little depression.

Supporting the Aged Person's Need for Mastery/Control. A sense of mastery or competence is significant to one's effective adaptation to the long-term crisis of aging. A sense of control or mastery over even a portion of one's life is a strengthening feeling, and, as such diminishes that most destructive of feelings, namely, helplessness. Loss of a sense of control or mastery over one's body or bodily functions can be one of the most degrading experiences for a person. Old age, illness, and disability rob us of a sense of control over our destiny. Indeed, nursing care often removes the element of control in decision making from the patient. The elderly have so many losses that they need to feel mastery over some part of their situation, if only on an intellectual level.